Triathlete EQ

Triathlete EQ

A Guide For Emotional Endurance

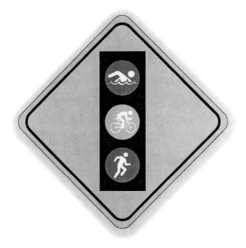

Dr. Izzy Justice and
Heather Gollnick,
5-Time Ironman Champion

iUniverse, Inc.
Bloomington

Triathlete EQ
A Guide For Emotional Endurance

iUniverse books may be ordered through booksellers or by contacting:

iUniverse
1663 Liberty Drive
Bloomington, IN 47403
www.iuniverse.com
1-800-Authors (1-800-288-4677)

ISBN: 978-1-4759-9282-3 (sc)
ISBN: 978-1-4759-9281-6 (hc)
ISBN: 978-1-4759-9280-9 (e)

Library of Congress Control Number: 2013909545

Printed in the United States of America.
iUniverse rev. date: 05/29/2013

About the Authors

Heather Gollnick is a professional triathlete, 5-time Ironman Champion, mother of three, and winner of over 200 multi-sport events, and currently resides in Steamboat Springs, CO. She is the President of GetFitFamilyRacing (.com) and IronEdgeCoaching (.com). Heather married her high-school sweetheart, Todd, and together they have three beautiful children, twins Josh and Jordan, and Zachary. Heather continues to dedicate herself to helping others reach their highest potential in sport, assisting her athletes in balancing all aspects of daily life, family, training, mental strategy development, and time management. Interested athletes can reach Heather through her personal website www.heathergollnick.com, or coaching website, www.ironedgecoaching.com

Dr. Izzy Justice is a sports neuropsychologist and an active age-group triathlete. He has worked with professional athletes, coaches, and teams in a myriad of sports. He was the first to formally introduce EQ to sports and is considered one of the pre-eminent experts in Emotional Intelligence, having published four books previously and in several sports magazines. He speaks globally on EQ and his weekly blog (http://izzyjustice.wordpress.com) is widely read. He and his family live on Lake Norman in North Carolina.

Dedication

To my best friend and husband, Todd, and my three beautiful children, Joshua, Jordan, and Zachary, who are my daily inspiration. *HG*

To Stephanie, Lexi, Hunter, and my eternal mentor, Gary Mason. *IJ*

Acknowledgments

This book would not be possible without the input of many good friends and collaborators. We want to thank Bob Babbitt, Blake Becker, Linsey Corbin, Ben Greenfield, Heather Jackson, Meredith Kessler, Andy Potts, Pip Taylor, and Chrissie Wellington. In addition, we are grateful for the support of writing and editing from Heather Sansbury and Anjum Khan.

Contents

Foreword

Here is the reality. When we decide to buy goggles, a wetsuit, a new bike, and some running shoes, the feeling is that the key to getting to the finish line of any triathlon is all about the physical training we put in. How much training can we jam into each and every day? With work and family, and our brand new dedication for this brand new sport, life becomes a non-stop hurricane of activity.

We know each and every split time for each and every swimming, cycling, and running session, but when we get to that starting line we are, oftentimes, an emotional mess. Physically, we feel like we have done the work, but emotionally we're drained, raw, scattered, and fragile.

The swim gets delayed a few minutes and we lose it. The water is choppier or colder than we thought it would be and we start to doubt our swimming ability. We get a flat during the bike or a cramp in the run and we give up. A lot of times we find ourselves defeated mentally and emotionally and not enjoying or savoring our tri-journey. More importantly, we can become a downer to be around for family, friends, and co-workers.

It's about time that a book like *Triathlete EQ: A Guide for Emotional Endurance* has come into our lives. Triathlon is the greatest sport around – and training for, and participating in, these events should leave you, your family, and friends exhilarated by the experience. For any triathlete, brand new or seasoned, I guarantee that reading *Triathlete EQ* will give you some awesome new tools to add to your transition bag so that every race and workout is a great one.

See you in the transition area!

Bob Babbitt
Ironman Hall of Fame Inductee
USA Triathlon Hall of Fame Inductee
Co-Founder, Competitor Magazine

Introduction

Triathlon is one of the fastest growing global sports. USA Triathlon (USAT) had between 15-20 thousand members between 1993 and 2000. In 2011, annual membership exceeded 150,000, with most of the growth coming from triathletes between ages thirty-five and forty-five. The Sports Goods and Manufacturers Association (SGMA) estimated that about 1.48 million people attempted their first triathlon in 2010. Several reasons exist for this explosive growth, from variety of training, to personal fitness, to camaraderie of group training, to accessibility to races, and to the sheer satisfaction of saying "I am a triathlete," among others.

Triathletes typically fit the "Type A" personality and when it comes to training, they take their preparation seriously and tend to enjoy it. In many cases, the training is both addictive and rewarding, complementing that personality of competing and chasing a personal record. Triathletes spend countless hours in the pool or open water swimming against the clock, on bikes navigating challenging terrain, and on the roads, trails, or track running to beat their previous times. A recent study showed that in addition to the sheer volume of time, they also spend an average of $4,500 per year on the sport between registration fees, equipment, nutrition, and coaching. The longer the triathlon, the more training time required, and concurrently, time away from other activities like family, friends, home projects, and other hobbies. Make no mistake — this sport requires a major investment of personal time and money.

Yet, despite the significant investment triathletes are committing to the sport, almost no time is dedicated to training for the one dimension that comes into play in all three facets of the sport: emotions.

The central premise of this book is that triathlons are as much an emotional endurance test as they are a physical ability test.

If you do not believe this, then this book will be of little value to you. If you do, then the next logical question should be: What do I do to prepare for the emotional endurance test?

The USAT estimates that less than five percent of triathletes spend any amount of time on training emotions and the resulting thoughts and monologues. Triathlons are an endurance sport, especially half and full distances or Ironman. It takes hours to both train for and compete in these events. During these long hours, the sheer volume of monologues that occur is quite unprecedented. Each monologue on any leg of the triathlon is a natural human response to the stimuli of the ever-changing environment. Whether it is other athletes swimming around you or the temperature of the water, riding through miles of roads in wind or heat or hills, or running on changing terrain, the environment in a triathlon is constantly changing and challenging. Compound this with the competitive environment of a race with other athletes, fans around you, no teammates or coaches to help you, as well as the myriad of things that can go wrong, and we are talking about a totally unique environment that will challenge your emotions to the core.

These emotions, both good and not so good ones, will dictate the tone and content of the monologues and critical subsequent decision-making. In Chapter 1, we will share several stories that almost all athletes will be able to relate to, where they had some issue in their own way, failed to execute their strategy for the race, and underperformed.

Yet despite powerful personal stories of underperformance and many more well-documented ones from professional triathletes, the average triathlete still spends almost zero time training his or her emotions and thoughts. We researched dozens of training plans for all distances of triathlons recently and found none that had budgeted time for this kind of training.

This is the reason we came together to write this book. We believe that most triathletes are grossly under-training in an area that has the potential to be a game-changer in performance. The inexplicable reason, we believe, that very established tri coaches and very intelligent and hard-working athletes are under-training in this area is simply that they do not know how to do it.

This book is not about swimming correctly, riding smoothly and efficiently, or running in perfect form, nor is it about equipment or nutrition. There are plenty of resources for these dimensions of the sport that are readily available. Triathletes are notorious for buying anything that they believe will make them perform better, but there is no off-the-shelf equipment for our emotions that can be purchased. This is a personal endeavor.

Heather Gollnick: As a five-time Ironman Champion and top 5 finisher in 18 other Ironmans, I have harnessed a wealth of practical knowledge that I use in my own training as well as with triathletes I coach. As a former competitive collegiate gymnast, I had to have strong mental focus to be able to flip and fly on a four-inch wood balance beam. I realized the mental strength I had as an age-grouper when I started triathlons was a huge advantage and I carried that onto over 200 multi-sport victories. I have won several races not because I was the fastest swimmer, biker, or runner, but because of my mental fortitude and ability to dig deep and fight both mentally and physically. I have made mistakes and had successes, and learned a great deal from both. I am excited to share them with you in this book.

Dr. Izzy Justice: As a sports neuropsychologist, I have worked with professional athletes, coaches, teams in many sports, as well as with business professionals for over two decades specializing in Emotional Intelligence (EQ). I have noted a profound weakness in the emotional literacy of people in general whereby most folks do not have sufficient knowledge of how to process emotions. Athletes, in particular, who are gifted physically in their sport, are even more prone to this weakness because they lack time for the deep introspection often required to learn and grow one's EQ, simply due to the fact that it often takes away from the physical training of their sport. As an age-grouper triathlete myself, I am proud to share in this book very practical information that will allow you to get the best out of yourself.

Together, we bring decades of experience and neuroscience. We hope this book will be an invaluable asset to both your physical and mental training, and the actual races. We will start the book with real-life stories and quickly proceed to why it is so important to master the art of learning from your mistakes in the sport of triathlon. Then we will provide you with detailed and easily understandable neuroscience of how the human body works; what emotions are and how they are created; how to recognize, label, and manage them during training, pre-race anxieties, and each leg of race-day. Each chapter will have both EQ and practical tips. Finally, we will explore recovery and life balance: two areas that we believe are also under-trained with roots in EQ.

Our goal is to not just give you tips to be a better triathlete, but to also help you understand why that tip will work for your body from a neuroscience perspective. This combination of knowledge is guaranteed to help you with your athletic goals, and almost surely, with your personal journey of growth as well.

What we provide you are essentially two books: one that we wrote, and the other written by you in the spaces provided within this book. Thus, if you do all of the written exercises we suggest, you will have a second book written by you, and for you. Either or both of these books can be read many times over during your season.

Emotional endurance is not just a part of triathlons but also a part of life. It can be argued that life itself is an emotional endurance test. And this may be what makes triathlons so popular, as you can draw parallels between training for, and participating in, a triathlon and your own life's journey. We hope that the reader-interactive format will impact both your physical and emotional endurance.

Chapter 1
Why train in EQ?

From Chrissie Wellington - World Triathlon Champion

In sport, we play with the mind as well as the body. Success rests, in part, with having the mental fortitude necessary to overcome our fears, hurt, and discomfort and cope effectively with the mental and emotional rollercoaster. This is part of training - the part that people don't put in their log books; the part that all the monitors and gadgets in the world can't influence or record. If we let our head drop, our heart drops with it. But if you can keep your head calm, focused, and determined then your body can be capable of amazing feats. Whilst some of us are born with that huge mental strength, it can also be learned and developed; and there are practical strategies one can use to train the mind - the most important weapon of all.

So why invest in learning about Emotional Intelligence (EQ)? We recognize that you are already spending hours on three different sports, transitions, nutrition, equipment, and recovery, so why add yet one more dimension to your training plan? Perhaps the best way to establish the case for this is to review several examples of what happens all the time in every race. What follows are actual stories shared by triathletes, professionals, and amateurs alike. We had literally hundreds to choose from but selected just a few that underscore the fact that mishaps are almost guaranteed to occur in a triathlon, and it is your emotional response to them that can be the difference between underperforming and recovering to overachieve.

"Winning isn't everything, but wanting to win is." - Vince Lombardi

Impact of Competitors

At an Ironman event, a pro-athlete was leading the race until about mile 16 of the run when another pro athlete passed him. He had led the entire race and was shocked to get caught. So disheartened by this, he decided to try to keep up with the new leader and go faster than he knew he could. Intellectually, he knew that he could not keep up the faster pace this late in the race but chose to ignore this and push himself even harder. By mile 22, he was spent and instead of a certain second place finish, he ended up twelfth. After the race, he was visibly upset. He just could not understand why he reacted the way he did when he got passed, why he abandoned his race strategy, and how he let his emotions at the time he got passed cause him to ignore his training, and instead adopt a totally unrealistic running pace. He clearly underperformed and it had little to do with his physical skills.

Impact of Changing Conditions

Another accomplished age-grouper athlete tells the tale of trying to make the US team in the ITU Long Course Nationals in 2010. On race-day, he woke to strong winds, which were not his favorite racing conditions. Shortly before the race was scheduled to start, the race organizers cancelled the swim resulting in a time trial bike start. Unprepared mentally, he ended up standing around for about 45 minutes, waiting for the race to start, and not knowing what to think about. His anxiety got worse and worse. He ended up not dealing with the winds well on the bike, not focusing at all on his strategy, and burned out before the run even began. To this day, he says that, mentally, he let the swim cancellation and winds take him out of the race before the race had even started. He was so well prepared physically for the race and believes that if he had mentally prepared for adverse events, too, then he would have qualified for a world spot. He clearly underperformed and it had little to do with his physical skills.

Impact of Anxiety

Yet another age-grouper tells us of how months of excellent training went to waste on race-day when her pre-race anxiety caused her not to sleep the night before – a common occurrence amongst athletes of all levels. She spent the entire night thinking about all the things that could go wrong and was a wreck before the open water mass swim start. She said she felt like throwing up and just did not want to be there anymore; her body felt about 25 pounds heavier, and her brain was filled with every negative thought imaginable, including mysteriously recalling that a man had drowned a few years earlier on that race. She started the swim and after getting bumped the second time, she waved to the kayaker and pulled out of the race. She was incredibly disappointed that all those hours of physical training had not prepared her for what happened on race-day. And worse, she still did not understand why it happened or know what do to. She clearly underperformed at her race and it had little to do with her physical skills.

"Never give up! Failure and rejection are only the first step to succeeding." - Jim Valvano

Impact of Experiencing Defeat

A marathoner was competing in her first marathon. She had a coach, trained well, and was set to run a steady ten-minute-mile pace to meet her goal of finishing in under four hours. She felt so good, relaxed, and confident that she started running faster at a nine-and-half minute per mile pace. Subsequently, she hit the wall and ended up struggling to make a four–hour, thirty-minute finish, well below her expectation. Disappointed but more motivated, she signed up for another marathon three weeks later. This time she went out at a ten-minute-mile pace, but suffered from lack of recovery between marathons and ran even slower, finishing near the five-hour mark. This was devastating to her emotionally. How could she train so well and still underperform? Having a strong competitive personality, she entered a third marathon and underperformed yet again as she ignored her recovery. This perpetuated a downward spiral of overtraining and eventual injury. Recovery, a critical part of triathlon training (which we will discuss at length in Chapter 9), requires a tremendous amount of emotional intelligence, which she did not exhibit. She gave into her instinctive reaction of wanting to succeed at all costs. She clearly underperformed and it had little to do with her physical skills.

Impact of Over Confidence

Another age-grouper, who had several half and full Ironmans under his belt, recalled doing a short sprint race that should have been a walk-in-the-park for him. It was a perfect race-day, and feeling incredibly confident, he began the open water swim near the lead. He said he felt amazingly comfortable, almost like he could swim all day without trying and was smiling. He recalls thinking he was not going to watch his competition, who were all behind him. Then suddenly, a boat approached him and told him he had missed the turn at the second buoy. He looked up and was way off course. He had mistaken a very distant buoy on the lake as his marker. So discouraged, he turned back and swam his lungs out in a manner that felt incredibly uncomfortable. Not making up much ground on the swim despite a valiant effort, he decided to hit it even harder (well above his FTP or functional threshold power) on the bike – after all, it was just 18 miles. He ended up walking much of the 5K. He said it was the worst piece of humble pie he had ever had, and for the life of him, just could not figure out how so quickly he went from a smooth swim on a perfect morning to a horrible race. He said afterward that had he just continued back at his normal pace, he would have enjoyed the race more and finished without bonking. He was just so upset about making such a silly mistake. He clearly underperformed and it had little to do with his physical skills.

Impact of Over-reacting

Norman Stadler, the Ironman World Champion, was competing in Kona as the defending champion in 2007. While on his bike, he experienced his first flat tire and started to visibly get upset. His entire strategy was built around having a huge lead on the bike, so when he had yet another second flat further down the road, he emotionally blew up. He was on the side of the road, very distraught. Furious with his situation, he threw his bike off the road — and the NBC cameras and the tri world were watching his meltdown! What had happened was that Stadler had not done his own bike prep; instead, his mechanic had set up his bike. The mechanic had glued the bike tires directly to the rim, so there was no room for Norman to use his tire lever to remove his flat. There were other options available, as we will describe later in how Chrissie Wellington responded to a similar situation, but Stadler had had enough. Once again, we see an athlete who let the emotions inherent in competition compromise his reaction. He clearly underperformed and it had little to do with his physical skills.

Impact of Nutrition

During an Olympic distance bike portion of a race, an age-grouper tells us of having worked hard with her coach on several calibration rides agreeing that she needed 300 calories per hour in order to have adequate calories for a successful race. After a smooth swim, she got on her bike and had one gel a few minutes later. When it came time for her next gel, she felt like she was doing just fine and did not need it. At the next gel time, she was down in the bars pushing hard and wanted to finish out a long flat straightaway, so she did not want to break that momentum and lose time by coming out of the bars and taking a gel and water. When she got to the end of the flat stretch, she felt like she should wait until she was done with the next hill, and then the next, and before she knew it, she had gotten completely off schedule and was way behind on calories. Though she had an excellent bike, she bonked just before mile 4 of the run. She did not understand how feeling so good could be such a bad omen and entice her to abandon her training strategy. She clearly underperformed and it had little to do with her physical skills.

Other Sports

Athletes from all sports experience similar mishaps, setbacks, and losses that are not attributable to the athlete's physical or technical skills. What must be noted in these other sports and athletes is that the common thread is how all athletes are first human beings built with the same physiology and neuroscience, and exhibiting the same emotional responses as triathletes.

➤ A basketball player practices free throws thousands of times, yet something is different when the free throw has to be made with one second to go and the game is on the line. What is different? Is it the size of the basketball? The size of the rim? The distance to the basket? Did the basketball player suddenly lose weight or get shorter or lose 20 IQ points? No, of course not. What is different is the pressure of the situation – the emotions of the situation.

➤ A professional golfer will tell you that there is a big difference between playing golf on a Thursday in the first round of competition and on Sunday, the last day of competition, as time is running out. On Sunday, the consequence of every shot literally translates to thousands of dollars. Again, what changed on Sunday? It was not the golf ball, his clubs, or the golf course he had just played the last three days. What was different was the pressure of the situation – the emotions of the situation.

➤ A NASCAR driver and his crew chief tell us that the race is called and the driver raced differently in the first 200 laps versus the last 50 laps. The difference between the winner and the next 10 drivers is literally seconds, so the last 50 laps are critical for finishing position. But the track is the same as it was in the first 200 laps. What was different was the pressure of the situation – the emotions of the situation.

> ➤ A professional tennis player tells us the difference between the first four sets and the fifth set is just one thing: mental strength. She says it almost ceases to be about tennis, and whoever can remain calm in the moment of pressure and execute the shots they know they have hit thousands of times before in the fifth set almost always wins. What is the difference between the sets? What is different is the pressure of the situation – the emotions of the situation.

It should be noted that there is a fundamental difference between these kinds of stories of underperformance and others where athletes underperform because of physical reasons. Getting injured during the race is one example of something that is physiological, not emotional or mental. When something irreparable happens to your body, no amount of EQ can compensate for that. If, for example, you sprain your ankle on a pot hole in the road during your run and you are in pain, good EQ cannot heal the ankle. Though still disappointed, most triathletes can live with these kinds of physiologically-based underperformances. It is the ones we have just been describing that are much harder to swallow because you feel it was something 'mental' and the root cause of your poor reaction is still inexplicably a mystery to you. In these underperforming situations, you feel like you lost control and let something derail you. You feel like you beat yourself. This is where EQ can make a tremendous difference.

"It's not the will to win that matters—everyone has that. It's the will to prepare to win that matters." - Paul 'Bear' Bryant

So Why Train in EQ?

As we've just read, triathlon races are littered with these stories of self-inflicted wounds where the mind chose to make poor decisions in the heat of battle and, in many cases, those decisions were contrary to what they and their coaches had already agreed upon during training. Why did their minds deviate from their strategy? Why did they react in a manner where in hindsight, and with a much clearer mind, they would have all made different and better decisions? What is it about athletes' emotions during anxiety situations that shut down very logical decision-making, decisions that they can make on any other day without blinking an eye? What could they have done during training to prepare them for the 'heat of the battle' scenarios?

As in all sports, if the athlete is able to maintain composure, access their training memories, and simply perform as they have trained, their chances of being successful go up significantly. *This is why we train in EQ.* We prepare ourselves to stay focused and positive in the midst of mishaps and distractions so that we can perform our best on the race course as well as in everyday experiences.

Our contention is that not only can these situations be managed differently during a race, but in fact, you can also effectively train for them and increase your EQ. It is impossible to predict what is going to go wrong and when it will happen, but suffice it to say, in all likelihood something will happen that will cause anxiety just before or during a race. This we can all agree on. And if you concede this, then in order to perform at your best on the day that it counts, your training plan must also prepare you to manage your emotions and thoughts. A plan that incorporates EQ training will help you manage the unpredictable, but certain-to-occur, anxiety-inducing experiences and your responses to them. As noted in the introduction, if you are going to spend so much time and money desperately searching for how to do a perfect race, why not spend just a few minutes a day to cultivate your EQ and remain positive and focused in the throes of situations that are beyond your control? No one wishes for chaos of any kind during a race, but a positive recovery from a bad situation can actually be incredibly motivating and powerful to spur you on to an even better performance.

"Competitive sports are played mainly on a five-and-a-half inch court, the space between your ears." - Bobby Jones

Please take a few moments to write down in your own words an experience where you underperformed in a race, similar to the stories shared earlier in this chapter. In subsequent chapters, as we share tips, we will ask you to come back to this story and personalize your learning. By writing down your own personal experiences, your own emotions and presence in the experience will make the learning and subsequent growth a much richer endeavor. As you write your story, try to describe yourself emotionally, mentally, and physically, as well as describe the situation you are in as graphically as you can.

Note that a mishap is not just a situation where something has gone terribly wrong (like a flat tire or losing your goggles), but it can be any circumstance where you have lost your focus, and as a result, deviated from your desired strategy or technical form and underperformed.

Exercise: My Personal Story of Under-performing

Top 3 Ideas
I learned from this chapter

1.

2.

3.

3 Action Steps
I will take immediately to incorporate the above
learning into my training and race-day strategy

1.	
2.	
3.	

Chapter Summary

1. Mishaps are bound to occur on race-day. They happen to all triathletes: professional and amateurs.

2. When mishaps happen, our emotions are tested. This emotional test is what most triathletes also need to train for.

3. When your emotional reaction to a mishap is poor, your decision-making is compromised and you underperform.

Chapter 2
Neuroscience of an Athlete

From Pip Taylor - Professional Triathlete

I am an athlete who feels the pressure when racing. All internal pressure I put on myself to meet my own expectations and sometimes this can be crushing. For me, being able to perform optimally is when I can put this aside, focus on the process and not the outcome, and do everything I can in that moment. This comes down to preparation in training, not just being confident of my physical preparedness and fitness but being able to visualize key parts of races where things may or may not be going to plan and being able to 'see', 'feel' and 'think' about how I will deal with these scenarios. In that way, when it comes to race-day, nothing is a surprise and you have mentally rehearsed those scenarios - both the good and the bad. Another aspect that I find critical is being able to relax and realize that I am actually enjoying myself - I love training hard and I love racing, and feel incredibly fortunate that this is what I am able to do - but sometimes it is easy to forget that in a race situation. Taking the time to breathe, relax, and look around is not only calming but reminds me that racing is actually really fun - and that reminder is a real performance enhancer!

It is critical that you understand how your body works physiologically. Your body is the ultimate equipment in your race. If you can shell out thousands of dollars on equipment like your tri-bike and spend hours riding it to figure out your optimal riding position, cadence, gears, wheels, watts, etc., then consider spending quality time on understanding your body as a piece of equipment that you need to appreciate with the same amount of passion and detail. Unlike the bike, however, your body (including emotions and thoughts) is constantly changing, which makes understanding it even more important.

For athletes, who measure success by their performance on each leg of a triathlon and how well all three sync for either a great race or better yet a PR, let us now analyze how all the components of the body 'equipment' fit together.

Superior Performance

The ultimate goal for you is to perform at your best on race-day. Period. Once you are physically ready (training), and as we discussed in many examples in Chapter 1, good and timely decision-making is at the heart of optimal performance, where you are able to perform those physical skills. Decision-making, therefore, is the centerpiece to optimal performance since without it, you are guaranteed to underperform. As shown below, superior performance is the end game with good decision-making at the center of it.

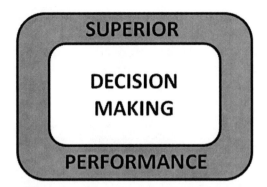

Figure 1. Superior Performance

Competency

The way that you know you are making good decisions during a race is directly related to your ability to execute your physical abilities, or competencies. Competencies or skills are the things you know how to do because of how you have trained. They are specific skills and abilities, such as the mechanics of your swim stroke, or your run form. Triathletes spend an enormous amount of time here. In other words, good training and technique play a big part in decision-making and subsequent performance. But most of you already know this.

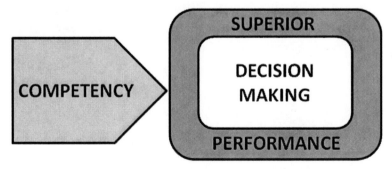

Figure 2. Competency

Behavior

Preceding our competencies and skills, are our behaviors. See below in the sequence of understanding how good decisions are made.

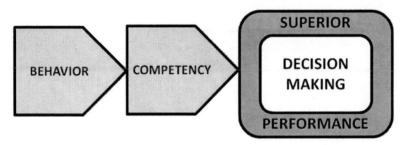

Figure 3. Behavior

Behaviors are essentially the framework of how we show our thoughts and emotions. For instance, showing the emotion of happiness by smiling or the emotion of anger by yelling — smiling and yelling are the behaviors we all know well. All of us know people who have mastered specific competencies in life, but some inadequate or inappropriate behaviors have diluted their competencies, which in turn, compromises their ability to perform at high levels. So these people, although full of potential, let their innate talent go to waste because of poor behavior. In triathlons, when things do go wrong, it is the responsive behavior that everyone sees.

Behavior is a response. Make no mistake about it. It is a response to your brain's interpretation of an experience. See Figure 4.

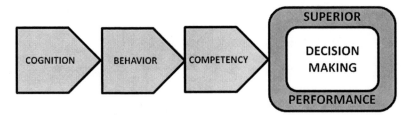

Figure 4. Cognition & Behavior

Cognition

Cognition precedes behavior. Slightly oversimplifying this concept, cognition refers to one's intellectual capacities, thoughts, knowledge, and memories. This is the rational part of our brain. In effect, it is our ability to take data points, weave them together in some cogent manner and reach a conclusion that dictates, consciously or subconsciously, what behavior to exhibit. If your thinking leads to the wrong conclusion, then the rest of the steps in the sequence to good decision-making will be compromised no matter how competent (skilled) you are.

"The spirit of sports gives each of us who participate an opportunity to be creative. Sports know no sex, age, race, or religion. Sports give us all the ability to test ourselves mentally, physically, and emotionally in a way no other aspect of life can. For many of us who struggle with 'fitting in' or our identity – sports give us our first face of confidence. That first bit of confidence can be a gateway to many other great things!" - Dan O'Brien

Emotional Intelligence (EQ)

What finally precedes cognition in this physiological sequence to high performance is your Emotional Intelligence (EQ).

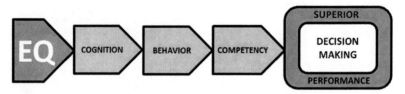

Figure 5. Emotional Intelligence

What you see in Figure 5 is the neurological sequence in human beings in all decision-making, whether it is athletic or in day-to-day life. Emotions are the first neurological response by your body—the equipment. Everything is dictated first by your emotions. Emotions lead to thinking which leads to behavior, which is the uniform you wear as you perform your skills. You can see how easily your skills could be compromised, especially in the heat of battle as they are so farther down the sequence. Skills stand no chance against the power of your emotions and how your brain is interpreting data especially in real time (race-day) when everything seemingly is at stake, and happening at warp speed.

Our five senses aggressively and constantly send signals to the prefrontal lobes of the brain located in our forehead area. This is the 'port of entry' of all stimuli. Everything we see, hear, feel, touch, and smell gets sent here for primarily one purpose: to assign a threat rating to that experience. Happening in microseconds, the higher the threat level, the more the secretion of powerful hormones like cortisol (fear), which can cause high states of anxiety. The lower the threat level, the smoother the transition into the subsequent steps of the diagram above allowing you to think clearly, behave appropriately, and ultimately perform to your best ability.

Neuroscience of "pressure"

"Adversity causes some men to break; others to break records."
- William Arthur Ward

The terms anxiety, nerves, pressure, stress, heat-of-battle, choking, being-in-the-zone, and the like, are used not only in all sports, but also in everyday life. Let us dig deeper into understanding our body, the equipment, in the context of these terms.

Our brain is the only place where all our cognitive functions reside. Cognitive functions include our long-term, short-term, and working memory. Put simply, the brain is our filing cabinet and command center. For example, if you have just learned how to run with a forefoot strike, that learning sits in your brain, not in your feet or legs. There is no such thing as muscle memory. Muscles do not have any memory cells or neuropathic abilities. You can train your muscles and body parts new motor skills, but in terms of the command to execute those new skills, that comes from the brain. A person in a coma whose body is perfectly normal is unable to perform any physical activity because the command center, the brain, is disabled. Everything you know and have learned is stored in the brain. This is a key point in the context of underperforming as athletes often wonder post-race why they made poor decisions or say in hindsight that they might have made better decisions.

From the command center, the brain, all orders are sent to different parts of the body. The body itself cannot do anything without the brain. The brain sends all its instructions through the spinal cord. In other words, the spinal cord is like a bundle of cables for that critical information from memory banks to be sent to parts of your body. Now, as shown in the following graphic image, conveniently located between the spinal cord and the brain (between the command center and cables) is the amygdala.

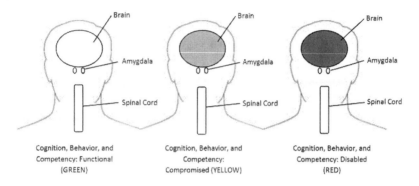

Cognition, Behavior, and Competency: Functional (GREEN)	Cognition, Behavior, and Competency: Compromised (YELLOW)	Cognition, Behavior, and Competency: Disabled (RED)

Figure 6. Impact of Amygdala

The Instinctive Emotional Response

The amygdala is a gland that secretes hormones in your body, as described earlier. It is situated there because its job is to respond according to the directions of the prefrontal lobes – the threat center. The prefrontal lobes sit in your forehead area. Within microseconds of sensing a potential threat, the amygdala releases hormones in your body that either partially or entirely disables your brain. This disabling of cognitive functions enables your body to respond quickly and instinctively to that danger. This is essentially a safety mechanism, which is triggered as a reaction to every threat, no matter whether the danger is perceived or real. Our bodies have spent thousands of years morphing into this state so that we can perform our primary function: recognize danger and react to survive. This is no different from most other living organisms. Although there are some universal physical dangers, such as someone pointing a gun at you, most emotional threats have no standards. It is different for everyone, and based entirely on our past experiences, often times from our childhood or previous failures.

For example, if you're crossing a road and you see a car coming at you from the corner of your eye, you would (without thinking) instinctively jump or run to get the heck out of the way. You would not think about it; you would not analyze, "I wonder how fast the car is going. What are my options here?" If you did that — if you used the cognitive functions of your brain — you wouldn't be able to respond fast enough and you would be hit. So the brain has to be disabled for you to instinctively jump out of the way.

Similarly, cognitive functions are disabled when triathletes get into situations that they perceive as danger, such as getting pushed at the start of mass swim start or other mishaps. The physiological response in the body after that push is virtually identical to that of a car coming at us. In other words, the amygdala does not make the distinction between the threat of a car coming at us and the threat of the consequences of a bad start or a flat tire, for example.

"Baseball is 90 percent mental. The rest is in your head." - Yogi Berra

Look at the body's physiological automatic and instinctive response to anything perceived as a negative experience, depicted in the following illustration. In this state, no athlete can perform at their best. In every race, as already discussed, the triathlete will be in this state. And even if something does not go wrong, body fatigue, hydration, and nutrition issues all force the amygdala to do its instinctive job.

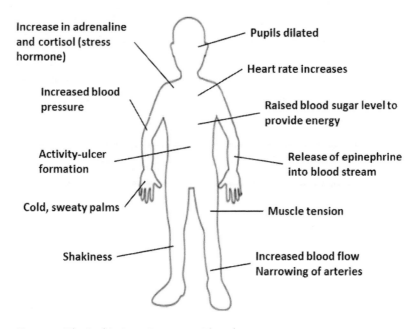

Figure 7. The Body's Auto-Responsive Physiology

This physiological state leads to a "high alert state" where the brain is operating in "lock down mode." The following consequences apply in this state:

- Decreased cognitive performance

- Less oxygen available for critical brain functions

- Tendency to over generalize

- Tendency to respond with defensive action

- Perceive small stressors as worse than they actually are

- Easily aggravated

- Recollection of past negative experiences

- Struggle to get along with others

- Cannot perform at your best

This state leads to those negative monologues, where we doubt our training, question our will, and recall past negative situations unintentionally. At that point, access to our rational ability and skill memory has been disabled and we are in the instinctive fight-or-flight mode. Again, no triathlete can perform their best in this state. They simply are hijacked by their own bodies in the most natural and instinctive of ways. It is a virtual guarantee that every triathlete will be in this state several times during a race. The question then becomes how to manage this state. This is where Emotional Intelligence (EQ) comes in.

"To succeed...You need to find something to hold on to, something to motivate you, something to inspire you." - Tony Dorsett

Negative Monologues

There is arguably no greater threat to an athlete than his/her own negative monologue. We all have them not just in triathlons but in life as well. You know the ones where you talk to yourself about all the reasons why you cannot or should not do something, where you recall the worse memories, and seriously doubt your ability to perform. There is no athlete or human being who actively pursues a negative monologue. They happen without choice, and very often, at the most inopportune of times.

Conversely, athletes often say that when they are at their best, in the proverbial zone, that there is no such negative monologue. In fact, the calm state is almost euphoric as though everything is exactly how it should be and you are performing magic.

In a triathlon, an endurance sport of many hours, you are certain to have both types of dialogues. We will discuss at length how to manage your emotions and these dialogues but it is important to understand how the negative ones, more harmful to your performance, are created.

Let us say you had ten experiences yesterday and nine of them were spectacular ones (very positive), but one of them was a negative one. For example, the negative one may have been you accidentally touching a hot stove and slightly burning your hand while making coffee. Today, the day after, which experience do you think you will be remembering more? If you answered honestly, then it would be the negative one. Why? Once again, our physiological design and construction from thousands of years takes center stage. Our brain has a specific place in the back of our skull where in fact negative memories are stored. When we have negative experiences in life, whether traumatic ones or like the slight hand burn, the brain needs to store them so that they can easily be retrieved. You NEED to remember the burned hand more than the nine positive experiences because the burned hand plays a larger role in your survival than your positive experiences. You need to remember to be careful next time you are near a hot stove.

In this manner, almost all of our life's negative experiences are not only permanently stored, but they are in fact the ones that are first retrieved if the prefrontal lobes (Threat Center) labels a current experience as a negative one (one with potential threat). So as the amygdala disables the brain in high anxiety situations after getting word from the prefrontal lobes, your cognitive functions are further limited to those negative memories and thus the negative monologues. In Chapter 1, the triathlete who was nervous at the swim start after a restless pre-race night mysteriously recalled of a drowning at that lake. This is because at the time she learned of the drowning, even though it was not her own experience, her brain still was on alert and doing everything to protect her even though the circumstances were totally different.

It is, therefore, very important for an athlete to take inventory of those past negative experiences so that he/she is, at a bare minimum, aware of what they are so he/she can anticipate the nature of the negative monologues should they occur. In this book, you will learn how to do this as well as how to proactively induce positive monologues during the race but more importantly, during those unpredictable mishaps.

Exercise: Your Negative Memory Bank

Make a list of the experiences of your life that you feel
are possibly stored in your negative memory bank:

1. _____

2. _____

3. _____

4. _____

5. _____

Exercise: Your Negative Monologues

Make a list of the most common negative
monologues you have with yourself

1. _____

2. _____

3. _____

4. _____

5. _____

Exercise: Your Positive Monologues
Make a list of the most common positive
monologues you have with yourself

1. _____

2. _____

3. _____

4. _____

5. _____

"An athlete cannot run with money in his pockets. He must run with hope in his heart and dreams in his head." - Emil Zatopek

How to increase your EQ

The first step in increasing your EQ is to learn to take your emotional temperature. Imagine an old thermometer, the kind you stick in your mouth. Imagine there are only three recordings it can give you – GREEN, YELLOW, and RED – similar to that of a traffic light.

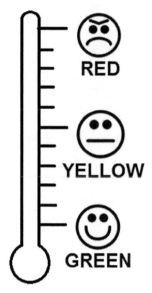

Figure 8. Emotional Thermometer

Green indicates that you are comfortable, happy, stress-free, and can think clearly and perform well. Now that you understand the neuroscience behind GREEN, you will note that the prefrontal lobes have sent a low threat level signal to the amygdala. This essentially means your brain, where all of the memories of your training and strategy are stored, can easily retrieve skills and make good decisions—the center piece of your performing at your best. It also means that the negative memories do not have to be accessed, which enhances your chances of being in a good zone, since only positive monologues occur here. GREEN is a good temperature reading. You can learn how to give yourself an accurate reading by referring to the diagram above showing the body's state when in the RED state. When GREEN, you will naturally feel relaxed, you will feel like all your senses are alert, you will naturally have positive monologues and recall positive experiences, you will remember all of your focal thoughts in all the legs of the triathlon, and you will feel like nothing can throw you off your game. Much of your training probably feels this way.

YELLOW temperature reading indicates that you are a little stressed and anxious. Something has gone wrong in the race but it is not fatal. You can get your goggles kicked off, swallow lake or sea water, drop a water bottle, get a leg cramp or blister – the list goes on and on of things that can go wrong that can take us from "GREEN" to "YELLOW". You are not in green for sure because everything just described in GREEN is not happening, but you are also not in RED where the consequences are very serious. In YELLOW, negative dialogues are occurring but you are able to recollect some positive ones too. It is an internal battle. Most of your race-day may feel like this.

RED is when you are implicitly or explicitly out of control, filled with anger and rage, or disappointment and frustration. You are filled with negative monologues, even being abusive to yourself and perhaps others around you like the volunteers. You are looking to blame someone, instead of finding a solution. You are frustrated that you cannot think clearly or remember much. This happens when the perceived threat is interpreted in your brain as fatal; at this point, you feel missing your goal is imminent and very likely.

You can see now why it is so important to know your EQ temperature during the race. The good news is that taking your emotional temperature is not something you can only practice in a race or during training. Remember how all decisions are made, not just athletic ones. Everything starts with emotions. So, no matter where you are or what you are doing, every three hours of a normal day starting today, take your emotional temperature and give yourself a color reading. Are you GREEN, YELLOW, or

RED? After about a week of this, start to do it more often, perhaps every hour and then start to do it during training and the race. We recommend taking your EQ temperature every 15 minutes during a race by setting an alarm on your watch.

You must become a master at taking your own temperature. You do not have a coach or team member out there during the race who can help you do this. Clearly, if you are GREEN, then nothing needs to be done mentally or emotionally. Just keep going and maintain your focus. But if you are YELLOW or RED, then something has to happen to get you back to GREEN as fast as possible. Research has shown that it is rare to go from GREEN directly to RED unless something very dramatic happens. Usually, we progress slowly into YELLOW without being aware of it, and stay in YELLOW for a while, at which point, nothing dramatic is required to elevate to RED since you are essentially a fuse just waiting to be lit. This is another common mistake many professional athletes make. They do not do enough when in YELLOW to get back to GREEN and often think they are mentally strong to go from RED directly back to GREEN. This can be done, but it is much harder.

Once you have learned how to take your EQ temperature, then and only then can you know how to regulate yourself back to GREEN. The things you would do to go from YELLOW back to GREEN are very different from the things you would do to go from RED back to GREEN. Not every mishap is a RED. Dropping a water bottle is very different from having a flat at mile 80 which happens to be farthest from the nearest aid station.

To state the obvious, the goal is to stay in GREEN as much as possible. Note that this is an emotional state. Chapters 4 through

8 will discuss very specific mishap situations in pre- race, swim, bike, and run, and tips (emotional and mental) to help with typical scenarios in these legs of the race. In this chapter, by establishing these GREEN, YELLOW, and RED standards, you now have a language you can use with your friends and coaches to help you prepare in a customized manner.

Changing your Emotional Temperature: GREEN TO GREEN

Our five senses are the only connection our body, the equipment, has with ever-changing stimuli of race-day. Every 15 minutes as you take your EQ temperature on race-day, and you are GREEN, then the goal is to stay GREEN proactively. When already in GREEN, the best way to stay there is to actively overuse your five senses. We call this macro and micro FOCUS, and will be discussed in further detail in Chapter 4.

You would be using your eyes, for example, to focus on the smallest detail of whatever is in front of you. If you are biking, it would not be just to SEE the other cyclists or the road ahead, but also to notice gravels on the road and trees or hills on the side. For FEEL, you would not just be feeling for the wind, but also the air around you at every turn and even the air coming in and out of your lungs. For SOUND, it would not be just listening for cheers from volunteers, but also to the wind or birds or other sounds you normally would ignore. For TOUCH, feel the energy transfer from your arms to the water, or the sense of your hands on your bike or your legs integrating with the pavement as you run.

Actively engaging the senses is a powerful technique, a way to stay in the proverbial present, and to keep your self-awareness at a high state of alert. Think about it: if you are this focused and you notice that suddenly, for whatever reason, you are not, then you know your emotional temperature has changed. Something has caused you to lose focus. It is hard to know you have lost focus if you never had it in the first place. We discuss focus in greater detail and how to use it in both training and races in Chapter 4. For now, learn to appreciate your five senses as a critical tool set in the equipment of your body.

"For me, winning isn't something that happens suddenly on the field when the whistle blows and the crowds roar. Winning is something that builds physically and mentally every day that you train and every night that you dream." - Emmitt Smith

Changing your Emotional Temperature: YELLOW TO GREEN

The absolute first thing to do when you take your EQ temperature and you are in YELLOW is to breathe. This might surprise you since you are probably thinking that you are always breathing – what is up with that? No. Change your breathing. Take a count (cadence) of how long it takes you to breathe in, and take another count of how long it takes you to breathe out in the same normal breath. For most people, this normal breathing count is anywhere from 2-5 counts in, and 2-5 counts out. Practice right now and increase your breath in to average about 25 and your breath out to average about 25 also. You can do this by simply taking in your breath slower and releasing your breath longer in a very controlled manner. When the body physiologically is in YELLOW, recall that one of the symptoms is increased heart rate and increased breath rate. A lot of oxygen is being channeled to other parts of your body in anticipation of having to 'jump to avoid the car' but it is your brain that needs the oxygen. Slowing your breath by actively counting 25 in and 25 out, will slow down your heart rate, even if just a little at first, and begin to disable the amygdala and enable the brain. You will recall it is only in your brain that all your skills reside. You need your memories of skills and what-to-do list. This kind of EQ breathing allows you to use some rational thought by putting the situation that caused you to go to YELLOW into context.

Abdomen, Chest, & Throat (ACT) Breathing Technique

During physical activity and especially during race-day, there are essentially three levels of breathing that occur. The first is breathing at the throat, T-level. This is typically short and fast breaths where the breath-count in and out is less than 2. The second is chest, C-level, where the breaths are inhaled chest-deep with breath-counts in and out between 2 and 10. The last is abdomen, A-level, where a long slow breath in, to the level your lungs feel like they are touching your abdomen, is followed by a long slow breath out.

During race-day, most athletes are breathing at the T-level. High anxiety situations also automatically trigger your body to the T-level of breathing. This is instinctive and in response to the higher heart rate, which itself is a response by the body to prepare you for survival. Unlike cognitive or brain activity, breathing involves a lot of body parts and muscles and therefore, can be controlled even after the initial burst of anxiety to T-level breathing. This is the reason why it should always be the first step in managing EQ, because it is one of the easiest things to do. Though A-level (abdomen) breathing is quite challenging during a race, your goal should be to always be breathing at C-level during a race, especially in times of challenging conditions (choppy waters, uphill or windy rides or runs). We also recommend attempting A-level breathing during "free speed" situations (swimming with current, downhill rides or run). As you are training or racing, keep track of what level of ACT (Abdomen, Chest, & Throat) you are doing and know you can perform best at the C-level, so adjust your breathing accordingly.

The next step is to create a YELLOW CARD. This card will change over time, and perhaps even several times over the course of a season. Let's create your personalized yellow card first and then we will talk about how to use it to change the temperature (after breathing) from YELLOW to GREEN. Answer the five questions below with just a few words that will instantly take you back to a very specific point in time and place.

Exercise : Your Yellow Card

1. When/where was the best race you have ever had? (e.g., 2010, 70.3 Augusta)

2. When/where was the best swim you have ever had?

---

3. When/where was the best bike you have ever had?
4. When/where was the best run you have ever had?
5. When/where was the best recovery to a problem in a race you have ever had?

Transfer these questions and your responses on an index card (for race-day) or perhaps on your iPhone (during training) so that it is portable and can be with you when you need it.

Just as negative and threatening experiences have dire consequences to the chemistry of our body as explained earlier, positive experiences have the opposite effect. They can give us confidence by releasing dopamine, the counter hormone to cortisol (fear hormone) and inspire us to perform better. Research shows that it takes an average of five positive experiences to dilute a comparable negative experience. In other words, cortisol is more powerful than dopamine. The problem during training, and especially during a race, is that we cannot predict when those positive experiences will happen, any more than we can predict when the negatives one will occur. However, we can be certain that it is very unlikely that the positive experiences will conveniently occur immediately as the negative one is happening so that they can counteract each other. This is where the YELLOW card comes in. These five experiences can be induced into your system. They are impossible to remember during a race as you have so many competing thoughts and priorities, and therefore writing them down before hand is necessary. Some triathletes write them down on their equipment, bike, shoes, or outfit. You will need this list to counteract the cause of what got you into YELLOW so you can get back to GREEN.

After your breathing, when in YELLOW, take a look at your YELLOW card however it is you have decided to craft it. Granted, this will be challenging during the swim and we have an entire chapter dedicated to this.

But when riding or running, when you read it, take just a minute to transport yourself emotionally to that great memory and remember what worked so well and what you are capable of doing. The breathing and the YELLOW card (which induces positive counter interacting experiences) will impact your prefrontal lobes, the grip of the amygdala, and allow you to do what you need to do to get back to focusing and to GREEN.

Take note that you are using both your emotions (by taking your temperature) and your thoughts first, prior to using your skills to get to performing at your best again – just as the sequential physiological model dictates.

If you look closely during races you will often see a small photo of someone taped to the top tube of a bike. Maybe it is a picture of a loved one that has passed away and when looking at it the individual receives inspiration that could carry them from YELLOW to GREEN. In other instances, it may be a picture of themselves when they were 50 pounds heavier or back when they were unhealthy or prior to becoming involved in triathlons. These pictures or mementos work in the same way and often times bring an individual's emotions from YELLOW back to GREEN.

Changing your Emotional Temperature: RED TO GREEN

When something terrible has occurred and you have taken your emotional temperature and diagnosed yourself as RED, the first step is again to immediately breathe in the same way as for YELLOW to GREEN. This will be a little harder to do but more important. Try your best to get to A-Level (Abdomen) of breathing. In RED, your breathing will be very intense (T-level), your heart rate very high, and your vision blurred, just to mention a few symptoms.

The process to go from RED to GREEN is similar to the YELLOW to GREEN transformation. We need to create a RED card but the content will be very different. You will still need to induce positive experiences but they have to be of a very different and very powerful kind.

My first Ironman race as a pro was in 2002 at Ironman Wisconsin. One reason I became a professional was because I wanted to do the Wisconsin race as that was near my hometown of Sussex. I spent the year training, going to Madison and working on the course, and was very confident going into it. I attended the press conference, which I was not invited to, but still went and listened. No one knew who I was. Listening to the pro women I still had belief in myself and that I could win. I registered and received my lucky number 33 and thought I was all ready. During the race I had a fabulous swim. I saw the top pro ahead of me and passed her on the bike with all media cameras on me now! I had a phenomenal bike ride but when I got off the bike, my legs hurt so badly that I couldn't run. I ran anyway but couldn't keep up, started walking and got passed. Half way, on the sidelines I saw my daughter and mother-in-law both in their wheelchairs screaming for me, and thought how awful that I was feeling sorry for myself for having aching legs. They would have given anything to walk just a mile. I ran over, gave them a hug and high five, and started running again with only their faces on my mind, and won the Ironman.

-Heather Gollnick

Heather's story above is very powerful and clearly was incredibly effective to get her from almost not finishing at the half way mark of the run, to winning the Ironman in 2002. You, however, may not have your daughter and mother-in-law in a wheelchair at your race, and do not need to, to orchestrate a similar transformation in yourself during a RED state situation. You can self-induce similarly powerful experiences by completing the RED card below. The RED card, unlike the YELLOW one, rarely changes and is used in those rare RED situations we all hope to not have.

Your personalized RED Card: Answer the five questions below with just a few words that will instantly take you back to that point in person(s), time, and place.

Exercise : Your Red Card
1. What are the first names of the most important people in your life?
2. What are the first names of your best friends – the ones that will be your friends for life?
3. When/where was the place you have been happiest in your life?
4. When/where did you do something for someone so powerful that it changed their life positively?

5. What are you most proud of in your life – an accomplishment not given to you that no one can ever take from you?

Top 3 Ideas
I learned from this chapter

1.

2.

3.

---

3 Action Steps
I will take immediately to incorporate the above
learning into my training and race-day strategy

1.	
2.	
3.	

Chapter Summary

1. Your goal needs to be to perform at your best on race-day. This means making good decisions.

2. The physiological sequence of making good decisions starts with our emotions, not our skills or thinking. Therefore, understanding emotions is critical to optimal performance.

3. All our skills are stored in our brain, and in no other part of our body. The brain can be shut off as an instinctive survival response to any danger, perceived or real. When the brain is disabled, then poor decisions are made.

4. Knowing your emotional temperature at all times of the race is critical to your performance. There are 3 EQ Temperature readings: GREEN, YELLOW, and RED.

5. The goal is to stay GREEN as much as possible during a race by using the ACT Breathing Model and your five senses to focus.

6. If in YELLOW or RED, use cards (or similar approach) to induce positive experiences (dopamine) to counteract the impact of any mishap (cortisol).

7. These techniques begin to lay the foundation of being a Triathlete with high EQ.

Chapter 3
Art and Science of Learning

From Meredith Kessler - 4 Time Ironman Champion

For us triathletes, a lot of what we do is trial and error by nature. There is no set guide to determine how your body will react in a full Ironman, no foolproof plan so you won't have stomach issues, or no magical formula to determine how much water, electrolytes, or nutrition to ingest. The way I have trained myself to learn from my mistakes is to remember the feeling when you fail to reach your goals and work to avoid this at all costs. It may have taken a good 30+ ironman races to figure this out but I'm delighted to say: better late than never! I will continue to learn going forward in nearly every race - it is a constant progression of learning from our mistakes.

Additional statistics of a typical triathlete from the USAT reveal interesting data. The average age of a triathlete is thirty-eight, with nearly 70% having a professional career making over $125K a year. Less than 20% of triathletes are under the age of thirty. This suggests a very mature and intelligent group of people who are triathletes.

Triathlons encompass not just the obvious disciplines of swim, bike, and run, but also several others in order to perform well. These include strength and flexibility, nutrition, recovery, transitions, race-day strategy, and equipment. Based on the distance and terrain of your triathlon, you and/or your coach will create a plan that calibrates all this to your ability and goals. The point here is that unlike single discipline sports, there is a lot more to learn, to master, and to manage. Being very good at learning itself is, therefore, another skill that triathletes often overlook, yet is very necessary to optimize both training workouts as well as on race-day.

Let's take two triathletes, Jill and Pam, of equal caliber, have the same coach, and who both had a two-hour swim workout yesterday. Both of them reported to their coaches, then tweeted and posted on Facebook to their tri-club friends that they had completed their lengthy swim workout. When the coach debriefed both Jill and Pam, she learned that these identical workouts were executed very differently. Pam was very focused, did each set specifically as directed and kept track of her times. Pam shared several observations based on this data with her coach to discuss potential changes. The ***purpose*** of the workout was met. Jill, however, was distracted. She had a project at work that was not going well and her mind kept wandering towards solutions for the project. While she completed all of her sets, her focus was on and off, and as a result, she was inconsistent in her performance. As expected, her follow up session with her coach was not very productive. It was hard for her coach to know whether any of the issues Jill had were related to the workout or her lack of focus. Jill's workout, though commendable for the volume accomplished, was not nearly as good of a learning experience as that of Pam.

We decided to include this chapter in the book because we believe that EQ comes into play in your ability to learn as well, not just to perform on race-day. We also thought it was appropriate given the demographics of the typical triathletes and the fact that there is actually a lot to learn in this multi-discipline sport.

In this chapter, we will explore the art and science of learning. The objective is to have you become very comfortable with making mistakes, especially during training, and then to be able to have a framework to process those mistakes into learning that can stick with you for future trainings. Learning from mistakes is an emotional exercise as much as it is a technical exercise. We have addressed the EQ component of being a triathlete, and we will address all the disciplines of a triathlon separately in the proceeding chapters; but we wanted to focus on the technical components of good learning in this chapter.

Learning can occur proactively, as demonstrated by Pam in the example above, where mistakes are induced. This can be done using a trial and error approach to figure out what works and what does not. Learning can also be reactive where the mishap occurs as a by-product of the workout or race, often unplanned, but equally valuable for learning.

Myth about Learning

There is a misperception about learning that has spread quite rapidly. It is from Malcolm Gladwell's 10,000 Rule from his book *Outliers: The Story of Success*, which, incidentally, we believe is a great read. Many coaches in all sports are convincing athletes that based on the research of the book, in which Gladwell has suggested that it takes 10,000 hours to fully learn a skill and become an expert at it, that volume exclusively is the key to mastery. This has resulted in very high repetitive and volume-based training in many sports, often at the expense of focused and learning-based training. In the example of the swim workout for Jill and Pam, clearly those two hours were not equal. In the same mode, it could be argued that it may take Jill several two-hour sessions to accomplish what Pam did in her one session.

What Gladwell actually said was that it takes 10,000 hours to be a phenom, of which there are literally only a handful of in the world; men and women who consistently perform at extra-ordinary levels and are often known by one name like Jordan, Elway, Mozart, Chrissie, Phelps, and Tiger. In triathlons, this applies to the less than ten triathletes within the professional ranks, which comprises less than 0.2% of triathletes.

We fully appreciate the need of distance and volume in training for triathlons, but the point worth reiterating here is that you must make a distinction in your training between 'logging in the hours' and 'training with a learning purpose.' We will show you how to do the latter in this chapter which will allow you to be a much smarter learner and triathlete, optimizing the limited time you have as a working professional.

In an interview that 2012 Kona Winner Pete Jacobs did with Bob Babbit a few days after winning, Pete described how it took him almost five years to stop making the same mistakes and become a better learner. He talked vividly about his first Ironman, doing very well in it, training harder for the same race the following year, only to finish an hour slower. Almost all professional triathletes will tell you that it takes many years to figure out how to train properly, and be a very good learner.

"I've missed more than 9000 shots in my career. I've lost almost 300 games--26 times I've been trusted to take the game winning shot and missed. I've failed over and over and over again in my life. And that is why I succeed." - Michael Jordan

Traditional Learning

Most of us have formally learned in the same general methodology. It was the methodology used in most schools at all levels across the world. In the broadest sense, the methodology is based on academic models of memory and testing. Information was given to you in a classroom or other setting, and then you demonstrated that you acquired that knowledge at that specific time period (for example, a semester) by answering questions during examinations. We concede we are over simplifying academia, but only to underscore the point that we believe learning has historically been very flawed. Traditionally, there is a significant time-lapse between learning and applying that learning. As children, that may have been acceptable, but for most adults today, it is not.

As an adult, you learn best at the "point of need". This means that if you are going to build a cabinet in your house this upcoming weekend, then the best time in your life to learn about building cabinets are the next few days just before the weekend. Could you have learned a few weeks ago? Yes. Could you learn a few weeks from today? Yes. But now is the best time to learn because you have a need this weekend that necessitates knowledge. Your emotions and appetite to learn are at a peak. In the traditional learning model that most of us have been taught, the need is a false need – it's an examination at a specified time in the academic pipeline – not a true application of what you have learned in the semester. Some estimate that people forget almost all the courses they took in college within five years of graduating, often because what they have learned in the five years *after* graduating was much more experiential and relevantly applicable to needs (job). For triathletes, the opportunity to learn in every training workout is not just a philosophical argument, but very much a real one.

Another reason we believe why traditional learning models are flawed is that they typically have been designed to fit only one style of personality and learning. Extensive research in adult learning over the past 20 years has revealed that there are, in fact, many styles of learning, with no one being 'better' than the other. The key is to find out what type of learner you are and then seek to do your workouts and learning in that modality. Given this, it is important for triathletes to find training plans and coaches that are flexible enough to match their style.

Learning Styles

According to Neil Fleming's VARK Model, there are several learning styles. It is important to know your style. Note that your style may vary based on the specific need you have, the urgency of that need, and the availability of resources to learn. The styles are:

- Visual (spatial): You prefer using pictures, images, and spatial understanding.

- Aural (auditory-musical): You prefer using sound and music.

- Verbal (linguistic): You prefer using words, both in speech and writing.

- Physical (kinesthetic): You prefer using your body, hands, and sense of touch.

- Logical (mathematical): You prefer using logic, reasoning, and systems.

- Social (interpersonal): You prefer to learn in groups or with other people.

- Solitary (intrapersonal): You prefer to work alone and use self-study.

Learning Agility

What is actually more important than knowing your learning style is to have the desire to want to learn all the time. This is called having *learning agility*. Triathletes who perform optimally have very high learning agility. They view almost all experiences as an opportunity to learn and in fact, embrace weaknesses or mistakes as *the* reason to train harder and more effectively.

Not just in the examples above, but also with other athletes in all sports, we have seen incredible transformation in athletes who previously thought they were the hardest working athletes in their sport only to realize that they had not been learning nearly as effectively as they could have been. So make a commitment to learn from every practice and race and apply it in your next experience. Let us show you how.

"Most people never run far enough on their first wind to find out they've got a second." - William James

Learning Methodology

There is both an art and a science to learning. In the methodology we recommend, there is a blend between the art and science as well as a key third dimension designed to make sure that once you have learned something, there is a process to then make it stick. We call this last step the 7-7 Rule.

The Art of Learning

The art is the emotional component that we have already discussed in Chapter 2. In both proactive and reactive learning, it is important to be in GREEN in order to learn. If you are YELLOW (as was likely the case with Jill) or RED (as was the case with Norman Stadler), then your learning is compromised before your workout even begins. The first step for Jill could have been to take her emotional temperature on her way to the pool and upon realizing she was YELLOW, to then read her YELLOW card to allow her to get back to GREEN before her workout. In addition, Jill may be well served to also have YELLOW CARD-LIKE focal memories during her swim with brief and intermittent breaks to review her YELLOW CARD. This is much better than just going through the motions of the workout that Jill ended up doing.

"A good hockey player plays where the puck is. A great hockey player plays where the puck is going to be." - Wayne Gretzky

The Science of Learning

Once in GREEN, then the science of learning comes into play for both proactive learning (planned experiences) and reactive learning (unplanned experiences).

Below is a very simple Five-Step general template that we encourage you to use dozens of times or for at least six months. This template has instructions for completions. There is a 'clean version' of the template that follows for you to complete and an example of a completed template provided as well.

Exercise: Learning Template Instructions

1. **Problem Statement:** Each learning can only have ONE problem. You cannot have two or more problems in one template. A common barrier to learning is the tangled up nature of how we think about a problem. In addition, the problem statement is brief and NO SOLUTION OR CAUSE can be part of this statement.

2. **Symptoms of Problem:** There should not be more than 3 symptoms and if there are actually more, then pick the top 3. In addition, each symptom should be described in less than 5 words.

3. **Potential Root Causes:** Each root cause must be directly related to the symptom. If it is not, then it is not a root cause. There should not be more than 3 potential root causes and if there are actually more, then pick the top 3. In addition, each root cause should be described in less than 5 words.

4. **Sources for Solution:** There should not be more than 3 sources and if there are actually more, then pick the top 3. In addition, each source should be described in less than 5 words.

5. **Potential Solutions:** Each solution must directly address the root cause in step 3. The only way to know this is to try the solution and see if an impact is made to the symptoms in Step 2. There should not be more than 3 solutions and if there are more, then pick the top 3. In addition, each solution should be described in less than 5 words. These solutions could be from one or more of the sources in Step 4.

Exercise: Learning Template

1. **Problem Statement:** _____

2. **Symptoms of Problem:**

   a. _____

   b. _____

   c. _____

3. **Potential Root Causes:**

   a. _____

   b. _____

   c. _____

4. **Sources for Solution:**

   a. _____

   b. _____

   c. _____

5. **Potential Solutions:**

   a. _____

   b. _____

   c. _____

Sample Completed Learning Template (Pam)

1. **Problem Statement:** My 100 yard time rose from 90 seconds last week to 110 seconds this week.

2. **Symptoms of Problem:**

   a. My time was 20 seconds slower.

   b. I felt slower, like I had extra weight on me

   c. n/a

3. **Potential Root Causes:**

   a. I was tired

   b. I was swimming using arms only

   c. I did not rotate as well

4. **Sources for Solution:**

   a. My coach

   b. Have Jill watch me for my body position

   c. Watch a You Tube video

5. **Potential Solutions:** (after talking to coach & Jill)

   a. Watch my head/legs to see if I was dragging

   b. Do some drills before the next swim focusing on rotation

   c. Measure stroke count for different 100 yard times

Professional golfers are some of the best learners of all athletes. They have a good bit of time between shots, and after they have hit a bad one, they have time to think about it and even discuss it with their caddies before the next shot. But more importantly, what they do particularly well, and you can see this on TV most weekends, is that they recognize that the *best* time to learn is right after a bad shot. This is in fact true for all athletes.

In our example, the best time for Pam to learn is within 24 hours of her swim. After this, research shows that the emotional state (art) has altered significantly, especially in training (not race) and you have moved on to other parts of your training or life in general. With so many stimuli, Pam's best appetite to learn, i.e., her learning agility, is at its peak immediately after her swim as she wrestles with why her swim time was higher. In this example, the first 4 steps could be done immediately. This is what makes a good learner. Our general tendency is to skip the first 4 steps and immediately get to the solutions. A hasty approach often results in poor learning, creation of additional issues, and most notably, reinforcement of all bad habits (remember what the brain does when with bad memories from Chapter 2).

"The secret of life though, is to fall seven times and to get up eight times." - Paulo Coelho, Alchemist

We recommend, as almost all professional triathletes can attest to, to make your training very focused and use the templates above to make learning an integral part of your training.

The 7-7 Rule

The 7-7 Rule states that in order to instill new learning, it has to be experienced in 7 different ways at 7 different times within 7 days. The 7-7 Rule is designed to help you make sure that new learning has the optimal stickiness factor, so that it can be imprinted and retrieved by your brain when it is needed the most. In the world we live in today, the sheer volume of experiences vying for mindshare is enormous. An athlete has to give performance learning an added and proactive nudge to make sure it gets imprinted. One of the 7 ways has to be a negative imprint. That is, it has to be the incorrect way of doing things, or simply put, your old way of doing things. The 7-7 Rule is based on three concepts that are being weaved together for the first time in this book.

Structure and Accountability

The first of the three is research done by Dr. Gail Matthews on accomplishing goals. Take a look at Table 1 below.

Table 1. Achieving Goal Success

	Group 1	Group 2-3	Group 4	Group 5
Think about goals	✓	✓	✓	✓
Write about goals	✗	✓	✓	✓
Share with a friend	✗	✗	✓	✓
Weekly **progress report** to a friend	✗	✗	✗	✓
Success Rate	43%	56%	64%	76%

Her study demonstrates powerfully the value of having structure and peer support in accomplishing desired goals. The more of both, the better the chance of achieving goals.

Kinesiology

The second concept is based on the neuroscience of kinesiology, the study of human kinetics combined with memory formation, specifically of new neuro-pathways (ways of thinking). It essentially suggests that while learning, and in order to create stronger imprints (new neuro-pathways) in our brain, all five senses (hear, feel, sight, smell, & taste) must be collectively involved in the learning. In other words, the more engaged and experiential your learning, the greater the probability of it sticking.

3-1 EQ Visualization Ratio

The third concept is based on the 3-1 EQ Visualization Ratio. This suggests that 3 EQ based repetitions (non-physical) is equivalent to one physical repetition of an exercise. For example, if you are lying in bed, and you combine powerful visualization with imagination to recall a new learning three times, it is as good to your brain as actually doing the exercise itself once. In fact, researchers at the Cleveland Clinic Foundation demonstrated that mental training alone can sometimes induce muscle strength.

It is often implied when using the term visualization that you are referring to the future. You are often told to visualize success, or a goal, or a desired outcome before it has happened. There are so many good quotes out there from inspiring people on the power of dreaming about something better in the future. This is all good. It is healthy to lie in bed dreaming about something you have not done, something you want to achieve, or something no one has thought of. The emotional power from these kinds of exercises is tremendous, often resulting in confidence, courage, and hope, which are priceless emotions to have during training and race-day.

Because the past is filled with both positive and negative experiences, unlike the future where neither has occurred, we tend to not visualize or dream about the past. It seems counter intuitive at first pass. Why waste time visualizing something you have already done? Well, we argue that visualizing something successful that you have already done is actually more empowering than visualizing something in the future where you have not done it yet. It is easier to visualize the past simply because you were there, you have all the details of the training day when you had an "aha" moment or events where you performed at your best. You know where you were, how it happened, who else was there, and how it felt like emotionally. The past seems to get a bad rap as a place where only bad experiences exist and as such, we forget what a great place it can be to give us confidence, courage, and hope. The 3:1 EQ Ratio is, therefore, a powerful tool that triathletes should learn as an integral part of training. On race-day, however, it is hard to visualize anything as so much is going on. This is why the information on your GREEN, YELLOW, and RED cards is all about data points from the past since they are so much easier to recall, than trying to visualize something in the future.

Let's go back to the workout that Jill and Pam had, and apply all three concepts to see how we can make learning stick. As a result of being a proactive learner and demonstrating high learning agility, Pam went back to the pool with Jill and almost immediately was told by Jill that her legs were way low and dragging her entire body. This made sense as Pam said she felt heavy and the drag had increased her 100 yard time.

Although learning has occurred, at this stage it is NOT complete. Too often, we find ourselves making the same mistakes and having to learn the same solutions over and over again. Just ask any coach and they will tell you that it takes a great deal of reinforcement and thus time, especially with brand new learning, to get them to stick. The root cause of this incomplete learning is that not enough has been done to reinforce the learning at the time it was best to reinforce it – which was during Pam's second workout.

Applying the 7-7 Rule

The 7-7 Rule states that in order to instill new learning, it has to be experienced in 7 different ways at 7 different times, incorporating all the 3 research-based concepts of the 7-7 Rule. So for Pam, she has to consciously practice those legs being up and not dragging in 7 different ways at 7 different times (one of them being consciously doing it the old way to remind her to feel what she does not want to feel) to make sure her chances of not reverting to dragging again are enhanced. As an example, here are Pam's 7-7 action steps:

1. Do sets with pull buoy to feel legs not dragging.

2. Do the first 25 of every set within a work out with a conscious focal thought of legs not dragging.

3. Purposefully swim with legs dragging for a short 25 or watch someone else in another lane who is also dragging to remember that is not what you want to do.

4. Have Jill verbally describe what she saw.

5. Practice consciously with legs dragging for 25 (incorrectly) and then the next 25 with legs in correct position to notice the difference in feeling.

6. Tell at least 2 people about what you learned and did to fix your dragging legs.

7. While lying in bed, visualize the practice session in the pool and imagine all the movements as though you are there.

You can see Pam has incorporated all three concepts in her 7-7 Rule. She really wants to make sure her legs do not drag anymore as it can cost her valuable time and more importantly, over-work her upper body and have a limited glycogen tank.

Obviously, these modalities worked for Pam but they may not work for you. You have to decide what you can do, based on your past positive learning, to make sure enough diversity is included that is personalized to your own style of learning to make it stick.

In proactive learning, which we recommend for ALL your workouts, it is much easier to implement both the learning methodology (i.e., the art and science of learning) and the 7-7 Rule if there actually is a purpose to your workout. Having a purpose almost always means having a way to measure your output. It can be time, watts, distance, stroke counts, average numbers, spikes in heart rate, etc. And if you have a PURPOSE for your workout, then you are inherently opening yourself up to learning, because if that purpose is not met, then something did not go right. This then gives you the opportunity to apply the learning methodology and the 7-7 rule to imprint the fixes you have to make. Remember, you want to have these learning experiences in practice, not during a race where, as we described in Chapter 2, all the elements create a very non-conducive learning environment and quite frankly, there isn't enough logistical time or venue to practice different solutions to a problem you have never had before. The cost of learning in a race can be very high. This is why we recommend you truly embrace making mistakes; when you make them, learn from them. And if you do that, then you are preventing the prefrontal lobes from sounding a compromising alarm in your brain which dilutes your ability to make the right decision.

"Success does not consist in never making mistakes but in never making the same mistake twice." - George Bernard Shaw

Complete Your Learning Template with the 7-7 Rule:

Exercise: Learning Template

1. **Problem Statement:**

   _____

2. **Symptoms of Problem:**

   a. _____

   b. _____

   c. _____

3. **Potential Root Causes:**

   a. _____

   b. _____

   c. _____

4. **Sources for Solution:**

   a. _____

   b. _____

   c. _____

5. **Potential Solutions:**

   a. _____

   b. _____

   c. _____

As practice, apply the 7-7 rule to your solutions above:

1.

2.

3.

4.

5.

6.

7.

Top 3 Ideas
I learned from this chapter

1.

2.

3.

3 Action Steps
I will take immediately to incorporate the above
learning into my training and race-day strategy

1.

2.

3.

Chapter Summary

1. Being a proactive learner can significantly improve the quality of your training and races.

2. Learning takes place best when there is a purpose and there is both an art and a science to it.

3. Everyone has a different learning style and should utilize that style to take advantage of opportunities.

4. Learning is only half of the equation to improvement. The other half is to make that learning stick by incorporating the 7-7 Rule.

Chapter 4
Workouts and Training

From Heather Jackson - Professional Triathlete

My emotions and mental imagery definitely play a HUGE role in my training and racing! I have a variety of different things that I bring into my head, or repeat over and over, or focus in on. Depending on what sport I'm training in, I mentally imagine that I'm one of the best in that sport. For instance, during a running track workout, I pretend that I am Allyson Felix running all out and going for the gold, or pretend that I'm racing against her in the gold medal round. I repeat things over in my head, "I can go harder than this! Pick it up, she's beating you!" Or if it's a swim set, I pretend that I'm racing Michael Phelps, or that I am him going for the gold. I am super competitive and would race everyday if I could, and so I mentally make all of my training sessions into a race, even if it's just in my head. On a hard bike interval, I try to push certain watts and pretend I'm racing Kristin Armstrong. In my head: "Really, that's all you can push? She held way more than that (watts) for almost an hour to win the gold!" And then I can pick it up a little more. Or I mentally imagine certain courses that I'm going to race, like Vegas 70.3 World Champs. The other day I had hill repeats and I just kept repeating "Vegas....Vegas.... if you get up this hill in under 60 seconds, you will win! Hurry up, you're not going to win at this pace!" I also have images of past coaches (ice hockey, or my track cycling coach) yelling at me, "Is that really all you've got????" And it makes me swim, bike, or run harder. I've worked with a sports psychologist in the past about avoiding the "negativity" in my mental imagery, but it seems to work for me. I find I can get to another level by imagining someone is challenging my capabilities.

We have introduced you to several concepts so far, most notably that of how your body functions, triathlete EQ, and learning. We have given you several tools to incorporate into your training program. In the next four chapters, we will spend time exclusively on race-day, where it matters the most. But before we go there, in this chapter we will discuss the hours of training and workouts you do and how EQ can be incorporated both in coaching relationships and training programs. Race-day lasts just a few hours, but your training consumes countless hours for months prior to it. Practicing EQ during training creates new neuro-pathways that during race-day, when you need them most, will not be new. Race-day should not be the place to try something new.

Most of you are not professional triathletes and do not have countless hours to train, or for that matter, the necessary hours to recover properly from hard workouts. Recovery is something we will discuss in detail in Chapter 9. You also do not have the 10,000 hours, or whatever the correct number is, to master all the disciplines of this sport. As discussed in the previous chapter, your ability to be very good at *Learning Agility* is critical to optimizing your learning and growth curves so that you can perform at your best on race-day. A central premise for writing this book was that we believed that most training plans were good but incomplete as they tend to focus on volume exclusively or intensity without purpose or EQ. We also believe that most coaches are very good but also incomplete in their coaching by not incorporating EQ into the training plans of their athletes. Our goal is to help both coaches and triathletes build EQ into training plans.

Recently I talked with an athlete I coach about his preparations for an upcoming Ironman. He was excited that he had completed a 5 hour ride. I asked him:

1. What was your focus?

2. What did you learn?

3. What did you practice?

4. What was the goal?

He paused for a long while and finally said (#1) I don't know (#2) not sure, (#3) Biking, (#4) the goal was to ride 5 hours. He could have learned so much more during this ride and could have answered:

1. Focused on my Ironman racing.

2. Learned that I needed to relax my upper body.

3. Practiced my nutrition strategy.

4. Goal was to have energy after achieving the 5 hours to give me confidence for the marathon after the bike.

-Heather Gollnick

It is our belief that workouts like the one above are all too common among triathletes. All of you could decrease your learning curve times quite significantly by building EQ into your training plans and workouts. Based on our clients, we believe 50%-80% of all triathlon training is often referred to as "garbage" hours where hours are logged in without any purpose or learning. We define a "garbage" hour of training (be it swim laps or bike/run miles) as an hour where there is no specific purpose or where focus is poor. Think of a run workout where the only metric of performance was either the distance or the hours. No other objective was set, or met. No learning occurred that could be transferred into either future workouts or on race-day. These "garbage" hours can be lowered when training in groups and even lower with a coach on hand. However, they can be reduced significantly by incorporating EQ.

We have broken this section into general and specific areas of triathlon training. As in previous chapters, there will be opportunity for you to be engaged with your own personal experiences (part of the 7-7 Rule) so that your learning can stick after you have read this book.

Finding the Right Coach

"A good coach will make his players see what they can be rather than what they are." – Ara Parasheghian

All triathletes can benefit from great coaching. Should you desire to work with a coach, finding the right coach is quite possibly one of the most important decisions you will make as a triathlete and will have the largest single impact in your *preparation* for your race. We understand that cost is a major issue as well as the availability of coaches in your area. But these are old barriers, as coaches are not nearly as expensive as you may think, and with technology advances, it is very easy to work with a coach from just about any part of the country or world for that matter. Technology allows us all now to connect in real time, send videos and pictures, and/or use software to track our workouts and have them viewable by just about anyone. Sometimes a more seasoned triathlete than you can act as a good coach as well. Thus, there are many alternatives to the traditional coaching models.

Make no mistake – having a coach is as much about the technical preparation as it is the EQ preparation. There are some priceless advantages to having a coach. Some of the reasons to work with a coach include:

1. Facilitating personal growth: A good coach will believe in you, build confidence, and inspire you to reach your personal best.

2. Building a right plan for you: Your body, your skill level, your motivators, and your goals are unique to you. A generic or group plan cannot possibly take into account all these key variables.

3. Fostering accountability: A good coach will also hold you answerable to your training, which is something we realize many people need, irrespective of learning or behavioral style.

4. Committing to their athletes: A good coach will listen to you and be flexible, knowledgeable, and secure enough to change with the feedback. They will support you every step of the way.

Exercise: Coaching Style

Think of someone who has acted as a very effective coach or mentor for you in sports, your personal or professional life. Make a list of the top 3 qualities of what made that person a great coach for you.

1. _____

2. _____

3. _____

Because triathlons are a multi-disciplinary sport, it is not unusual at all to have several coaches, one for each discipline, and yet another for your overall training plan. It is also common to have coaches who are good at two of the three disciplines but not at all three. Many triathletes often see one coach more frequently than another based on their weaknesses or focus area at different points of the season. The point here is that unlike single discipline sports where there is one coach and one skill to learn, triathlons are much more diverse in skills, and thus, trickier to find coaches. But for reasons already shared, we strongly recommend a coach. More importantly, we recommend that you have a coach for the entire season so that you can build a collaborative relationship in an environment that promotes continual learning. Consider having one coach as your main coach throughout the season, and additional discipline specific coaches as warranted based on your deficiencies. If you are getting better each year, consider it quite normal that the coach who helped you get to this level might not be the right coach to take you to the next level, and thus finding a new coach once you have seen a plateau in your training and race results is something to consider.

> I believe that coaching an athlete goes far beyond the type of workouts; intensity of swim, bike, run, and duration or frequency of workouts. Although these are certainly important, an athlete will respond differently to the same type of stimuli (workouts) depending on their life circumstances. As a busy mother of three, fitting in training was not always easy. I like to make sure I help my clients find balance. I like to be the positive cheerleader and hard-line coach as needed, but you must be flexible and find that balance, what works for one does not work for all.
>
> *-Heather Gollnick*

Here are some general qualities to look for when finding a good coach:

- Is knowledgeable about all three disciplines and a proven expert in at least one of the disciplines

- Can build diverse and custom training plans

- Has the structure to hold you accountable

- Can adapt to your learning style

- Will build EQ and mental training into your plan

- Will listen, respect, and inspire you (you can initially assess this by speaking with other athletes they have coached)

Look at your criteria of a past effective coach and blend them with ours to find a right coach for you. Your training starts here with this very important step.

"Do you know what my favorite part of the game is? The opportunity to play." - Mike Singletary

Clinics

A very useful, cost-effective alternative to personalized coaching is to attend training clinics. Many retail stores and triathlon clubs often hold clinics throughout the year to support and engage community members. Clinics provide an opportunity to learn from other knowledgeable community members. This is, in itself, a form of coaching. From learning to change a tire to a video swim or run gait analysis, clinics can be a great way to learn at an affordable price.

Training Plans

As you prepare for your upcoming triathlon season, it is important to put together a training plan. Almost all of the training plans that we have seen start with a base period followed progressively to more demanding and intense workouts before a taper just prior to race.

Recently a highly motivated "Type A" triathlete (yes most are) I coach did not want to take recovery or any downtime after his session. For that matter, this same athlete did not want to have any weeks to build his base. In an effort to help explain to this athlete my line of thinking, I used the following word picture. I started by saying, hold your hands 3 inches apart. If your base is this big, I explained, then bring your hands together, forming a peak like triangle upward then your peak will only be this high. Now repeat this same exercise. This time hold your hands out about 12 – 14 inches apart. Now bring your hands up high – into a peak. Wow, look at the difference of how high your peak can be. You need to build the base then explain the reasons behind it to add value. Once an athlete understands, "Why" you build your base or "Why" you need periodization in your training or "Why" the taper helps you perform best, they open their mind to understanding and then incorporate it willingly into their training. Understanding is knowledge and knowledge is KEY!

-Heather Gollnick

There usually is a healthy balance during each week between hard workouts, easier low intensity ones, and recovery days. These variations in intensities are important. Table 2 below is a generic example of the first month of an Olympic Distance Training Plan.

Table 2. Sample Generic Training Plan

Month 1							
Week	Mon	Tue	Wed	Thu	Fri	Sat	Sun
1	30-Swim 60-Bike	Off	40-Swim	30-Run	90-Bike	Off	45-Run
2	20-Swim 45-Bike	Off	40-Swim	35-Run	90-Bike	Off	45-Run
3	30-Swim 60-Bike	Off	45-Swim	30-Run	90-Bike	Off	50-Run
4	20-Swim 40-Bike	Off	30-Swim	20-Run	60-Bike	Off	30-Run
Note: Time is listed next to each activity							

What we like about this training plan is that it gives appropriate volumes of effort each day, provides a recurring sequence of disciplines each week, and has built in recovery days. But what it lacks is flexibility and guidelines for intensity, the latter of which is discussed below under Specific Goals. In terms of flexibility, what about when you have a sick child and can't do the swim workout or run the following day? What if the weather is not conducive to your planned bike ride and you don't have access to a trainer? Do you jam missed workouts all into one day? Under these types of plans how do you, as an athlete, understand the real purpose of each workout? So even though plans like the one above are a decent starting point, they often times leave the athlete with more questions than answers.

Incorporating EQ into Training Plans

Here is how we recommend you build EQ into your training. The good news is that building EQ into your training does not add more hours to your current training volume. We recommend building EQ directly into the workouts you are already doing. Do keep in mind that the ACT Breathing Model discussed earlier applies to workouts.

Every workout must incorporate the following EQ-based dimensions:

1. Focus

2. Having a SPECIFIC goal for workouts

3. One SKILL FOCAL THOUGHT

4.   One EQ FOCAL THOUGHT

5.   Learning

Let us review these individually:

1. Focus

Focus during workouts can be challenging for all athletes, especially age-group triathletes who often are mentally preoccupied with balancing so many other important dimensions of their lives. Even for professional triathletes, quality focus can be intermittent during workouts. Focusing should not be confused with general EQ and the use of YELLOW and RED cards. Those are designed specifically for when something goes wrong. Focusing is irrespective of whether there are any mishaps or not; it is necessary for all athletes in order to optimize their learning and performance.

Our own rule of thumb is that for every time during practice that you find yourself not focusing, one out-of-focus moment (irrespective of how long that moment was) translates to 30 seconds of lost performance time. For example, in the one hour swim that Pam and Jill had in the last chapter, let's assume Pam counted 30 times during the hour that she was out of focus. These were times during swimming when she realized she was not focusing and just going through the motions. This cost her 15 minutes of swim time compared to Jill. In other words, if both had swum the same way in competition, Jill would be out of the water 15 minutes before Pam. This rule-of-thumb, by the way, applies to the bike and run portions of training and race-day also. Focusing is, therefore, a critical part of efficient racing - which arguably is what every triathlete wants. It starts in training though.

Here are two ways to get and stay focused during workouts. This approach, incidentally, also will work on race-day.

    a.   Macro Focus: is an emotional and mental transition from your regular life and chores to your life as an athlete who is on his/her way to a training workout. It is based on the cognitive supposition that *a conscious effort to think about one thing is a subconscious effort to not think about another.* We use this premise with athletes in all sports as they enter their arena for practice or performance. It uses all 5 sensory organs to be truly present in your workout. If, for example you are beginning your bike ride, then visually, force yourself to look at details of what is around you - everything from the trees, clouds, cars, etc. Start to notice them. Your conscious effort to notice them is a subconscious effort to not think about the list of worries or tasks you have to do. Use your ears to hear sounds. It is amazing how much you can hear on a bike ride if you consciously choose to listen to all the sounds of cars, wind, birds, people outside, etc. Start to feel your bike using your hands, feet, and gluteal muscles. Feel the energy you are exerting with all three. Taste intimately whatever it is that you are drinking or eating. Take advantage of this mundane and routine activity to feel the fuel entering your body and finding its way into your body. Smell the aroma of the environment that you are riding in. Proactively use your sensory organs for exactly what they are designed to do. By sensing the environment you are in, you are focusing on your arena by concurrently not thinking about competing thoughts that are not related to your workout. Obviously, you do not have to use all five of your senses at the same time, and use them as you find yourself losing focus on your workout. Macro focus is a low intensity emotional and mental effort that is easy to get into and stay in your arena, i.e., your workout, and thus, should be used as often as possible during all your workouts.

b. Micro Focus: unlike macro focus, micro focus is very intense and requires more emotional capital. As such, it should not be used very often and saved for those days when there is just too much noise in your head, and you feel like you are just showing up for the workout to go through the motions. It should not be used for more than just a few minutes interspersed with the macro focus that you should also be doing. But just like the purpose of RED card to jolt you back to GREEN, micro focus, too, can have the same impact regardless of whether there is a mishap or not. Micro focus is similar to macro focus in that you are using all five senses again, but the difference is that you only use one sensory organ at a time and take the focus of that one sense very deep. Instead of just looking at the tree, you are now focusing deeply at a leaf on the tree noticing every nuance of the color in it. When you listen for sounds, pick one and try to exclude all others so you can follow that sound for as long as you can. When feeling your hands on the bike, or water while swimming, feel your fingers and every part of what they are touching. When you taste your drink or nutrition, do it slowly so that you can feel your tongue and teeth working. This deep focus will allow you to return to your arena so that you can optimize the impact of your workout.

"Play like you are in first; train like you are in second."
- Fuzzy Minnix

2. Specific Goals

All your workouts in your training plan must begin with focus. If you have no focus, then the rest of the components of building EQ into training become compromised.

Once you are in your arena, and fully present to work out, then the next step is to have a goal for that workout. As we discussed in the last chapter, if you have a goal, then you open yourself up to learning. With a defined goal, you will know during your workout whether you are meeting it or not. If you are, great. If not, then there is an opportunity to learn. Goals also allow you to know whether you are focusing or not. If, for example, the goal of your workout is to run at a certain heart rate zone, then monitoring your heart rate zone requires focus during the run. What is the point of this workout if you forget to look at your HR zone until the end of the workout? Goals allow you to learn proactively since your ability to meet that goal or not will be a valuable source of learning. As we have said before, better to have this learning in training than on race-day.

In the sample training plan, the only goal is time. This is not a bad goal as much as it is a very one-dimensional plan. This is where a coach can be very helpful to you so that you can bring in other goals into your training, and thus, you have more areas of learning opportunity. If you only measure time, then your learning will be limited to just that. We recommend you and your coach blend in other goals including:

   i.   Heart rate zone

   ii.   Power meter zone

   iii.   Distance

   iv.   Distance *and* time

   v.   Drills to focus on deficiency

   vi.   Stroke count in swim

   vii.   Tempo times

   viii.   Cadence

   ix.   Pace

   x.   Pace *and* heart rate

   xi.   Perceived Exertion (PE), recovery heart rate, or recovery intervals.

The second step in incorporating EQ into your training plan is to have a very specific goal for each workout. By having a goal, you are setting yourself up for learning since you have set a metric to measure your performance. Learning, as we have discussed already, is key to optimizing your innate skills.

Exercise: Your Specific Goals

Write down some specific goals for your workout next week:

Swim WO Goal: _____

Bike WO Goal: _____

Run WO Goal: _____

"Setting a goal is not the main thing. It is deciding how you will go about achieving it and staying with that plan." - Tom Landry

3. Skill Focal Thought

Once you are focused and have a goal for your workout, then it is time to focus on building your skills and becoming a better triathlete. That is the objective of training, right?

A focal thought is one specific skill base form or technique that you can use in your workout. For example, in swimming, it might be the entry point of your recovery arms; for bike, it might be the exertion point of your stroke; for run, it might be the strike position of your foot. Whatever the skill focal point is, it must be very directly related to something you and your coach are working on. It usually is a thought that helps you remember something that you are just learning or often forget to do. Every workout must have at least one skill focal thought. It should be used throughout your workout, and this is where your ability to focus (macro and micro) can really help you master this skill focal thought.

Exercise: Your Specific Focal Thought (SFT)

Write down some specific Skill Focal Thought (SFT) for your workout next week:

Swim WO Goal: _____

Bike WO Goal: _____

Run WO Goal: _____

"All that we are is the result of what we have thought." - Buddha

4. EQ Focal Thought

A great example of focal thought is visualization. As an example, when I go out for a training ride I visualize my competition. My training partner often times may be a male, but I see him with a pony tail and as someone I want to stick legal distance behind for the next 20 miles, then I want to make my move and pass her (actually him)! One time, a few years back, I was so into training visualization exercises that I even called my male friend and training partner by a female competitor's name!

-Heather Gollnick

Similar to the skill focal thought, an EQ focal thought is much simpler. It is an EMOTIONAL focal thought. It usually is just one word or a very short phrase for that specific workout. Its purpose is to get you to relax and even enjoy your workout. It may be the name of your collegiate mascot, your favorite pro triathlete, the race you are training for, your spouse or children, your favorite color, or anything that works for you.

Exercise: Your EQ Focal Thoughts

Make a list of all the EQ Focal Thoughts that come to mind and use them for your workout next week:

a.

_____

b.

_____

c.

_____

d.

_____

e.

_____

f.

_____

g.

_____

h.

_____

i.

_____

j.

_____

"Everything you need is already inside." - Bill Bowerman

5. Learning

One of the best ways to optimize your training workouts is know when it is the best time during the workout to learn and to apply all the concepts discussed. Whereas learning itself can occur any time and at any place, we submit that the best time to learn, apply, and test your race-day strategy, especially when it comes to focus, is the last 25% of your workout, regardless of duration. In other words, whether you are swimming for 30 minutes or 2 hours, or biking for an hour or 4 hours, or running 3 miles or 20 miles, the last 25% of these times and distances is the best time to learn and apply focus and focal thoughts. This is because the last 25% of your workout is when you will be most tired, most distracted (lack of focus), most depleted of nutrition and hydration, and most likely to underperform by reverting to poor technique or abandoning your strategy. See the depiction below and etch it permanently in all your workouts. Make the time to practice more on micro focus and your combination of EQ and Skill focal thoughts during this last 25% and you will see a tremendous improvement on race-day.

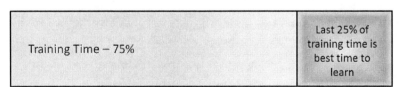

Figure 9. Optimal Training Time

We also recommend that every single training workout end with using the Goal Post Model.

New objective/ goal achieved (lesson learned)

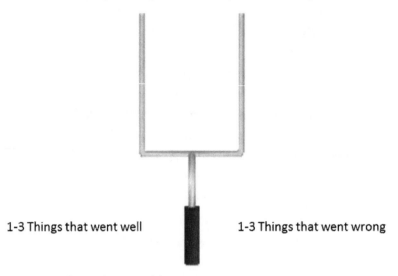

1-3 Things that went well   1-3 Things that went wrong

Figure 10. The Goal Post Model

The Goal Post Model is quite simple. As you can see in the picture, the goal post looks like a tuning fork. After every training workout, simply draw the goal post in your note book. Write down on the bottom left side of the post, just 1-3 things that went well in the workout, and on the bottom right side of the post, 1-3 things that did not. Then on top of the goal post, write down what you learned and/or might want to do different for the next workout. This should be based on your original goal of the workout. Do this immediately after your workout and review it just before your next training session whenever it may be. This model converts mundane and long training workouts into a learning activity, and allows you to have a goal for your the next session. It is that simple.

If you stumble on something you cannot figure out in training, then use the model in the previous chapter to do a deeper analysis of what you need to learn.

This is the last step in incorporating EQ into your training plan. Remember, it is better to learn during training than on race-day. If you are focused, then you can have a goal that you can test in training. If you have a goal, then you can know whether you have met it or not. This in turn sets you up to be a very good learner.

As a coach, I deal with athletes on many different levels. With beginners there is so much to learn, and they are like sponges. With these athletes, the rapid improvement is exciting for any coach. Then you have athletes that follow your instructions to "T" (love the student pets!).

I had two women who trained together almost daily for their first Ironman. They followed the plan along with nutrition and mental prep guidelines that I devised for them exceptionally well and as a result they both experienced great success and are now Ironman vets!

We have talked a lot about learning and the hardest thing for a coach is when an athlete does not learn. Many times it is the athlete that has the most natural talent that will not put in the time or effort to learn, thus never fully reaching their potential or goals.

I am very specific with certain key workouts I give as to the "goal" of the session. When an athlete's goal is to nail his/her nutrition and the athlete calls half way through the brick that he/she is "bonking," I go through a checklist with them to help. But the athlete who forgot to eat or didn't bring any nutrition can be very frustrating. Yes, I have traveled to train only to arrive and realize that I left my water bottles on the kitchen counter as I ran out of the house. But most certainly the next week, I double and triple check so it does not happen again. I have bonked so bad (years ago) that I "learned" and now never bonk. I not only carry enough food/nutrition for myself but for all my training partners as I hated the feeling and don't want to see anyone else repeat it ever again.

-Heather Gollnick

Having a skill focal thought and an EQ focal thought will eliminate other variables in order to truly measure your physical ability to meet the established goal. If you have met the goal, reward yourself! If not, reward yourself again with the realization that you have just discovered an opportunity to be better! You win either way! What could be better?

Learning is the only additional time that would be added to the sample training plan. All the other steps of incorporating EQ are integrated into your workout, so it is not an additional time requirement, yet allows you to have a much more productive workout.

"Tell me and I forget, teach me and I may remember, involve me and I learn." - Benjamin Franklin

Top 3 Ideas
I learned from this chapter

1.

2.

3.

3 Action Steps
I will take immediately to incorporate the above
learning into my training and race-day strategy

1.

2.

3.

Chapter Summary

1. You can decrease your learning curve times quite significantly by building EQ into your training plans and workouts.

2. The best time to learn during a workout is the last 25% of the workout. This is the time to practice micro focus and focal thoughts.

3. Athletes who treat workouts as learning environments, with specific goals, focus, and learning (Goal Post Model), become more efficient and perform better on race-day.

Chapter 5
Pre-Race Strategy

From Blake Becker - Professional Triathlete

I think that it's been important to understand that our thoughts in life, while training and racing, only have meaning if we grasp onto them and give them meaning. We tend to ride the wave of positive thoughts, but then go into crisis mode when we get the smallest amount of negative feedback. I worked a lot with the four focuses (broad and narrow, internal and external). For me, the following things have helped the most: (1) Recall what it feels like to ride powerfully even if I am not riding well. I find that this helps me come around faster; (2) On the run I focus on a few keys within my run form. Usually relaxed shoulders and weighted elbows; (3) I have a mental plan going into each race. This is just as important as a nutritional or pacing plan; (4) I have a specific routine that I follow at every race; and (5) I consciously think: "I'm not attaching" to any negative thoughts that come into my mind.

The 24 hours leading up to the swim start, along with the hour just before, are quite possibly the most emotionally mismanaged time often causing incredibly high levels of anxiety. Many triathletes are in YELLOW or RED (EQ Temperature) before the race even begins. Though this is common in any competitive environment in all sports, and therefore widely written off as 'just normal jitters,' there is much that can be done to help manage the situation and your emotions.

No matter how well prepared you are, as we noted in Chapter 1, both age-groupers and professional triathletes are likely to experience some form of a mishap during race-day. This you can expect. Remember, a mishap is anything that derails you from performing at your best, which sometimes is a major issue like a flat tire but more frequently, is simply losing focus due to minor unplanned circumstances. What you do not know is what the mishap will be, and when it will happen. In Chapter 2, you learned to deal with the EQ dimension of the unplanned disaster, but what about the technical side of the mishap? Are there some practical tried and tested strategies that more experienced triathletes do to help them manage themselves not just in the 24 hours leading to the race, but also during each leg of the triathlon?

In this chapter we will address specifically the typical mishaps that can occur prior to the swim start. In the next three chapters, we will dedicate each chapter to race-day swim, bike, and run mishaps to help you have both an EQ Plan for them and techniques that professionals use.

"Success is going from failure to failure, without loss of enthusiasm."
– Winston Churchill.

Below is a list of very common mishaps that can happen before the race begins. Regrettably, one or more of these will likely happen to you on your race-day. It is better to have thought through (beforehand) how you will address the calamity during training.

As you review this list, make a note of how you will address them if they were to occur to you. You may already know how to address some of them, but may not know how to address others. The only way to know for sure that you are prepared is to address them in training or a previous race. If you do not have the knowledge or skill to address the issue, then work with your coach, peers, retailers, tri clubs, or seek out information from the internet (YouTube is an excellent source of "how to" information) and try it in training. Your candor in this exercise will only serve you well.

Potential Pre-Race Mishaps

- Fatigue due to poor tapering or overreaching due to anxiety (too much training up to event)

- Fatigue due to lack of sleep

- Upset stomach

- Inability to have a good pre-race meal

- Worrying about having all the right equipment

- Realize you have forgotten/lost an important piece of equipment

- Late for the race

- Unable to go to the bathroom at race site

- Forget to get a key race-day required activity (such as body marking or chip pick up)

- Forget to stretch or warm up before swim start

- Over-hydrate with water, diluting electrolyte balance

- Did not prepare for changes in weather (rain, colder or warmer than forecasted, etc.)

- Unable to find training partner, coach, or family member

- Getting stung by a critter

As a professional triathlete, I have had the opportunity to travel to many remarkable places including Switzerland, Dubai, Hawaii, Chile, France, and Austria. Travel is hard in and of itself, but when there is pressure to perform and your gear doesn't show up that usually means STRESS. One year when defending my 70.3 title in Pucon, Chile, my gear did not arrive for days and it was a major stress as it related to my preparations.

I was lucky to be able to borrow goggles and a run outfit to get some pre-race workouts in, but after that trip and ever since my dear friend Marc Strickland taught me a lesson on packing, I will never make the same mistake twice. Now I have LEARNED and pack ALL my race gear in my carry on! The items I will wear race morning and all my race gear I will need race day (minus the bike) to include; race shoes, glasses, goggles (two pairs, smoke and clear), mental script for race-day, any notes, affirmations for race, race belt, visor, nutrition, bike shoes and training outfits. If my bike does not come, I can always get one (not ideal) but to have to find bike shoes, get cleats adjusted and wear them in for race-day – that's a tall order. Now I just carry it all with me and it's much less stressful.

-Heather Gollnick

Make Lists

The easiest way to not forget something is to make a list. Period. You should create your own race check list with your coach, get one online or from a seasoned triathlete friend, and modify to meet your needs. Most lists capture just technical parts of the race, but a good race-day check list will include all the EQ ideas that we have been discussing in this book.

Below is an example of a well-balanced race-day check list that an age-grouper we work with used recently. Pay extra attention to the EQ prep and application. If you create a list like this, you will be able to address many of the typical pre-race mishaps.

Sample Pre-Race Checklist

General Prep

- Eat breakfast and adhere to pre-race nutrition plan

- Dress for race (trisuit)

- Put on Garmin watch

- Put on Road ID

- Apply Bodyglide

- Apply sunblock

EQ Prep

- ○ Practice maximum-count breathing

- ○ Visualize the perfect swim start

- ○ Playlist of 10 good monologue topics

- ○ Pack YELLOW card

- ○ Pack RED card

- ○ Listen to favorite playlist on iPod

- ○ Begin positive monologues and dialogues

- ○ Pack a GREEN card reminder (e.g., family picture)

Race check-in and transition set-up

- ○ Get body marked

- ○ Pickup timing chip

- ○ Take note of where you are in transition as it relates to swim finish, bike start/finish, run start

- ○ Check air pressure in tires

- ○ Check breaks on your bike

- ○ Reset computer, power meter

- Check that your bike is inappropriate gear

- Fasten race numbers to helmet and bike, if required by race

- Set up towel and transition gear as appropriate

Swim Gear

- Goggles

- Spare goggles

- Anti-fog solution

- Cap

- Body glide

- Sunblock

- Wet suit, if legal

Bike Gear

- Bike shoes

- Bike nutrition

    - gels, shot blocks, etc.

    - water bottles

- o   stinger waffles

- o   Helmet

- o   Sunglasses

- o   Socks

- o   Bike jersey, if needed

- o   Arm/leg warmers, if needed

- o   Bike gloves, if needed

Run Gear

- o   Run shoes

- o   Race belt

- o   Hat/visor

- o   Gels, shot blocks, etc.

EQ Application throughout Race

- o   Take EQ temperature

- o   Begin to use cards if necessary

- o   Think of swim/bike/run monologues or theme

○ Practice Macro Focus

○ Hear your favorite song in your head

And, don't forget to thank as many race volunteers as you can!

As a side, if you are traveling by air, pack the gear that you *will not* find at a local shop or expo at your destination, and take with you as carry-on luggage.

A girlfriend of mine was competing in a popular triathlon while wearing a wetsuit for the first time. Living in Florida, the need for wetsuits is rare. This triathlon, however, took place in the Midwest and I recommended that she get used to swimming in a wetsuit as it can feel very different. Because of the warm weather in Florida, she never did get used to wearing it. Race day came and it was the second time ever she had it on. The gun sounded and she was off. Very soon into the race she began to panic as she gasped for breath, feeling constricted in the wetsuit. She stopped and held on to a lifeguard paddle boat trying to regain her composure. Watching her competition fly by, she resumed swimming only to feel the same claustrophobic sensation and anxiety return relating to her ability to breathe. She stopped again and flagged down a lifeguard. As he approached, she decided to take off the wetsuit while in the water. She struggled as she bobbed up and down in the water trying to shed the wetsuit. Finally, she threw the wetsuit into the lifeguard's boat and struggled through the remainder of the swim. She didn't stick to the power outage and Heart Rate we had decided was optimal, as she felt the need to "make up time for her poor swim." The end result was a run/walk and overall disappointment. Her race experience that day was ruined because of her inability to prepare properly for the feeling of swimming in a wetsuit. As athletes we usually feel as though we are strong enough to overcome or fight through our troubles on race day. But the re-occurring theme that we will continue to hammer home in this book is PREPARATION – both physically and mentally.

-Heather Gollnick

Technical Mishaps

Half Ironman Utah (no longer on the circuit) - It was a half ironman that I was looking forward to racing and had prepared as an "A" race on my schedule. There were a lot of my new sponsors there as well. The pressure was on but I was ready. I had a great swim and got out of the water with the second pack and started flying on the bike and then I got a flat tire. I calmly changed it and got going again re-passing a few women that passed me while changing my tire. I was in the groove and going again then BAM... I got another flat. This one fixed, I kept going and got a third flat tire- who carries 3 spares? Man, I had to now wait, each minute seeming like it went on forever. Everyone passed me. All the age-groups passed me by as well. At this point I told myself I can either see this as glass full or glass half empty. So I took the positive road and started cheering for people. Race support gave me a whole new wheel, but I wasn't even in the pro race anymore because I was so far behind. It was a two loop run course and everyone was cheering for me because they thought I was in first place. Truth be told at this point I was getting lapped by the first place women. I stopped and ate so that the first place women could keep going. Along the journey I encouraged a 50 year-old man. I was not racing at this point so I kept encouraging the 50 year old man to push himself forward. I finished and went to look at results because I wanted to see my swim time. When I got to the front I heard a woman say, "Hey Bobby look, I out biked Heather Gollnick by 10 minutes!" But rather than feel dejected, I reminded myself that I cheered on the 50 year-old man who won his age-group and later gave me a big hug and thanked me for my help and encouragement.

-*Heather Gollnick*

Technical mishaps cause anxiety. They could be related to equipment, logistics of the race, or an accidental last minute mishap. This is where you need to work with your coach and peers. For each of the pre-race mishap we have listed, you must have already rehearsed the mishap during training and have a plan for it. If you show up on race-day in transition and realize you forgot your running shoes at home or the hotel, what are you going to do? If you know there are never enough bathrooms near the swim start, what are you going to do? If you cannot find the nutrition you swore you put in your bag the night before, what are you going to do? If the line to the bathroom is just too long and you have to go but there's less than 5 minutes to your swim start, what are you going to do?

Thinking through these and practicing them, if possible, can be just as valuable a part of training as all your hours in the pool, on the bike, and running, as they can severely impact both your EQ (required for the race) and physical ability to get started in the right way. Having rehearsed these mishaps and potential solutions also, from a neuroscience perspective, dilutes the impact of the prefrontal lobes. They would still label the mishap as a threat should it occur on race-day, but instead of labeling it as a RED, it might get a YELLOW rating, which is a lot easier to manage than a RED situation. The lobes will give this lower rating since it is processing an experience that you are prepared for.

Fatigue

Race-day fatigue can occur for many reasons. If it is because of lack of proper tapering, then it is very manageable. As noted in Chapter 4, a good training plan will have a built-in taper before your race. We strongly recommend that you strictly follow the training program, especially the taper. If you are working with a coach, all coaches should understand the need for tapering, and the issue usually rests with you, the triathlete. It is very difficult for many of you to taper. The notion of working so hard for so many weeks and months and then just as you are about to race, to significantly cut down on training seems very counter intuitive. What if my legs are not fresh? What if I lose my stamina? What if I forget my form? These are common fear-based (emotion) questions of self-doubt. Recall from earlier chapters that these negative monologues are based on fear (cortisol), the most powerful of all emotions because its central function is to keep us alive. Since this is quite possibly the last emotion you want to have going into the race, many resolve to overcome this fear by continually training hard during the last weeks before race. This is where your EQ can really help you manage your fear by diluting it with learning practices and the 7-7 Rule to imprint a sense of trust and confidence in your training, coaches, and widely-accepted advantage of tapering.

Fatigue can also set in because of lack of sleep during the nights leading up to your race. Though common, this too, is a manageable challenge. The anxiety of a race is very powerful. It is filled with excitement, the presence of so many other athletes in the area or at your hotel, and the anxiety that all your training will now be tested. This is all EQ related.

What we do with our athletes on the 2-5 days before the race, when in full taper mode with very low volumes, is substitute the physical training time with EQ training time. If you are up at night and not sleeping, then work on your EQ. Here are some things you can do several days prior to race:

- Practice taking your EQ temperature every hour

- Make current your YELLOW and RED cards

- Practice using your cards

- Engage in conversation with people who you know will be encouraging and have positive dialogues

- View every experience as one that can make you GREEN or YELLOW. By taking your temperature, proactively steer yourself toward GREEN experiences and steer away from YELLOW experiences

- Fine tune your suggested monologues for the race, and practice them on your taper days

- Begin Macro Focus through the week so that on race-day, you are already used to it

- On the night before the race, if you are not sleeping, then instead of letting your thoughts wander, engage in very strong visualization exercises where you recall past good races or past positive experiences of your life (in sport or life in general)

- Also, if you get up very early and want to do something, then practice light meditative yoga, using very low intensity poses in conjunction with light soothing music and practice A-level and C-level breathing in the ACT Breathing Model.

- The golden EQ rule is to engage in positive activities, the kinds that make you feel very good about yourself - that cause you to smile, laugh, and be joyful.

Fill EQ Tank during Tapering

One reason that tapering is so difficult for many is that it is emotionally counter-intuitive to slow down days and weeks before a race, especially after months of progressive increase in physical activity and intensity. To not feel the physical fatigue, sweat, soreness, and satisfaction of working out before a race is an emotional challenge. During tapering, we recommend substituting the hours of physical exercise with hours of EQ exercises. The goal is to enter the race-day with your EQ tank full and almost overflowing with positive feelings and thoughts.

This means to associate yourself with people, in activities and in experiences, who are very positive and encouraging. It also means to consciously avoid people and experiences that can be EQ depleting.

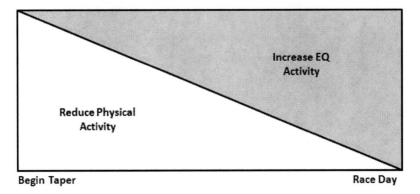

Figure 11. Taper Week: Volume Shift from Physical to EQ

Complete your taper week exercises below.

Exercise: Your Taper Week Activities to Fill EQ Tank

Make a list of 10 Activities you can do during Taper week that can fill your EQ Tank. These can be anything from watching your favorite movies, reading inspiring books, eating foods you love, talking to people who will be supportive, etc.

1. _____

2. _____

3. _____

4. _____

5. _____

6. _____

7. _____

8. _____

9. _____

10. _____

Exercise: Activities To Avoid During Taper Week

Make a list of 5 Activities to avoid during Taper week. You know from past experiences that these will deplete your EQ Tank. These can be anything from negative people in your life, to activities that are stressful, or events that require significant amount of your EQ.

1. _____

2. _____

3. _____

4. _____

5. _____

In working with other professional athletes who have major tournaments only a handful of times, this is the same kind of emotional preparation done during the week leading to the major event. Emotional nourishment during taper sets the stage for high EQ during the race. In addition, it addresses so many very manageable pre-race anxieties by filling the void of not logging in training hours.

Complete your pre-race mishaps exercises below.

Exercise: *Your Potential Pre-race Mishaps*

Make a list of 10 pre-race mishaps that could happen to you. For each one, think of a solution. Then, during training, purposefully induce one or more of these mishaps and see if your solution would work.

1. Mishap: _____

   _____

   _____

   Solution: _____

   _____

   _____

2. Mishap: _____

   _____

   _____

   Solution: _____

   _____

   _____

3. Mishap: _____

   _____

   _____

   Solution: _____

   _____

   _____

4. Mishap: _____

_____

_____

Solution: _____

_____

_____

5. Mishap: _____

_____

_____

Solution: _____

_____

_____

6. Mishap: _____

_____

_____

Solution: _____

_____

_____

7. Mishap: _____

_____

Solution: _____

_____

_____

8. Mishap: _____

_____

Solution: _____

_____

_____

9. Mishap: _____

_____

Solution: _____

_____

_____

10. Mishap: _____

_____

Solution: _____

_____

Top 3 Ideas
I learned from this chapter

1.

2.

3.

3 Action Steps
I will take immediately to incorporate the above learning into my training and race-day strategy

1.

2.

3.

Chapter Summary

1. No matter how well prepared, both age-groupers and professional triathletes are likely to experience some form of a mishap during race-day. What separates you from the competition is how you handle it.

2. The easiest way to not forget something is to make a list. A good race-day check list will include all the EQ ideas that we discuss in this book. If you create a list like this, you will be able to address many of the typical pre-race mishaps.

3. It is common to feel anxiety during your taper week. A good practice to help alleviate this anxiety and fill the void left by your decreased training load is to increase your EQ activities as you want to enter the race with an overflowing EQ Tank.

Chapter 6
Race-Day Swim

From Andy Potts - Olympian, 70.3 World Champion

I use the same mental approach to each discipline within the sport. The way I figure it, if I can do it in the swim then why not on the bike; if I can do it on the bike then why not on the run... you get the idea. I like to think that the mental game can transfer into each leg of a triathlon if you train for it. I train my brain just like I would train my arms, legs, lungs, and body. I like to break down long workouts into manageable parts. Once I have gotten over a stumbling block or a hurdle I can then tell myself, 'You've done it once, now all you have to do is do it again, 11 more times (or however many reps I had planned)'.

Specifically, the mental approach for swimming all starts with technique. There is never a shortage of things for me to concentrate on while training or during a race. A few things always seem to come back to me time and again, and that is to keep my fingertips down and my elbows up. Trying to make each stroke count so it will get me to my bike is the fastest and most efficient way to swim. Don't get overwhelmed with the big picture. Try to focus on the obstacle in front of you and stay in the present. Objective number one is get to the next buoy, and then reevaluate when you get there what the next objective is. Keep it simple and allow your training to come through without your head getting in the way.

111

The swim start of triathlons and the swim leg of the triathlon are probably the areas that give most triathletes anxiety. Unfortunately, there is some disturbing evidence to support this. According to the USAT, deaths in triathlons are twice as high as in marathons and virtually all of them occur in the swim leg, and mostly by drowning. There are obvious reasons for anxiety associated with open water swim. It is the start of the race, possibly the most crowded point of the race, usually in dark waters with limited visibility, and there really is no aid station or place to stop, stand, and take a breather as there is while riding or running. In other cases, it is because it is logistically harder to get practice time in open water swim than it is in a pool. Whatever the reason is, and given the personal risk involved, it is important to understand your anxiety at this stage, and have explicit EQ strategy for it.

I was conducting a training camp for Ironman Louisville. Swimming questions came up immediately for two main reasons; the time trial start and the current. We were at the river as a group when one athlete commented "doesn't look like much of a current today." We got in the water at point "A" and while we treaded, I explained how we were going to swim to another point "B" and back. By the time we were done talking we had drifted 15-20 feet from where we entered the water. As it turned out, there was a current and a strong one at that. This ended up playing a big role in developing the strategy on race-day for my athletes and how exactly they were going to deal with their anxiety of fighting the current. Where would they line up? If swimming into a strong current on race-day, how much energy do they expend? It is important as an athlete to have developed a strategy in your mind for dealing with open water swims.

-Heather Gollnick

Potential Swim Mishaps

As we did in the previous chapter, it is worth making a list of all the mishaps that could potentially happen during your swim. Here are some common ones:

- Unable to manage anxiety (high heart rate)

- Getting bumped and hit by other swimmers

- Getting goggles kicked off

- Water seeps into goggles

- Going off course (poor sighting)

- Swimming at a faster pace than you planned thus using more energy than planned

- Lack of focus, resulting in poor technique

- Unplanned head current or choppy water

- Getting stung by water critter

- Too crowded at swim start, resulting in poor start position

- Panic attack in middle of swim, not knowing how to handle it

- Wetsuit is chafing or too constricting

"The man who is swimming against the stream knows the strength of it." - Woodrow Wilson

Anxiety

One thing I find funny about myself is my race-day nerves. After over 15 Top 5 Ironman finishes you would think I'd have it under control… nope, not fully – however, over the years I have learned to compensate for the nerves. After I won my first Ironman (IM Wisconsin), I felt a target on my back. Soon after Wisconsin, I was competing in the inaugural Ironman CDA. I was ready! I got there a few days early, scouted out the course, my preparations went fantastic, my taper had gone well and I was ready to peak. The morning of the event I was so nervous, tossing and turning through the night, up at 4:00am, nauseous and could barely eat a thing.

By the time I got out of the swim and 5 miles into the bike I had been up and burning calories 3+ hours and I was bonking! I ate almost everything I had brought for the bike portion and had to use what was on the course to supplement my nutrition. Thankfully, I ate enough to come out of my bonk and have a super ride and run – ultimately going on to win my second Ironman.

To this day, before some events, I get so nervous that I actually dry-heave. Once before a race, as my husband and I were walking to transition (the day before!), I started to dry-heave and his concern was– "OH are you feeling sick?" I laugh now knowing it was nerves and it goes away when I think positive. On race mornings when I do a pre-race swim or jog, it all comes together. My pre-race mantra is "It's ok to have butterflies as long as they all fly in the same direction."

-Heather Gollnick

We have discussed how the brain works, the impact of a threatening stimulus and how it would cause your prefrontal lobes to sound the "alarm" to your glands thus disabling your brain and body. It is your perception of threat that is at the heart of your anxiety. This results in going to those negative memories and monologues, like the story we shared in Chapter 1 of the triathlete who carried her pre-race anxiety into her swim and underperformed.

We have shown in Figure 7 in Chapter 2 how your entire body reacts when in YELLOW, or under anxiety. One of the measurable symptoms is a very high heart rate (HR.) Research has shown that the first spike in anxiety (HR) is always the highest. This is why many times the first few hundred yards of the swim tend to be the most difficult, from an EQ perspective. The graph below shows a normal anxiety pattern. Over time, after the initial shock of stimuli alerting you to the start of the swim, your brain begins to note that nothing fatal has occurred and you can do this. You begin to 'settle down' as they say. Your anxiety (HR) is still high and spikes perhaps every time you look up, have a negative thought, or a mishap occurs.

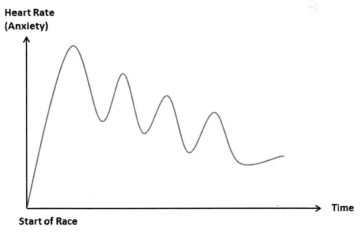

Figure 12. Normal Anxiety Graph

Knowing that, although to varying degrees, all of us are going to experience that initial spike in HR, one of the best ways to manage this swim start anxiety is to simulate the high HR just minutes before the start of the swim. See the graph below:

**Heart Rate
(Anxiety)**

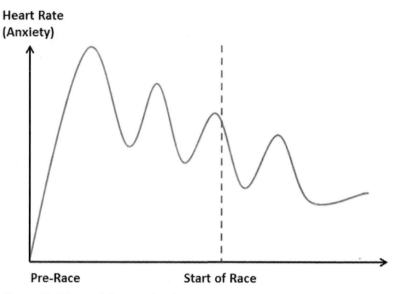

Pre-Race   Start of Race

Figure 13. Managed Anxiety Graph

In this graph, note that the anxiety levels are identical to the one before. The only change is in the horizontal axis where something has been done to experience the initial spike, which can be hard to manage amongst the chaos of the horn blowing for swim start. How can you do this?

"Effort only fully releases its reward after a person refuses to quit." - *Napoleon Hill*

The first step is to fully execute your pre-race strategy as discussed in the previous chapter. If you commit to filling up your EQ tank in the days leading up to race-day and having all the items checked off, your anxiety spike will be lower than if you run to the swim start knowing there are things that you needed to do but did not get to.

The next step has to be done between 5 and 15 minutes prior to the swim start, not any sooner than that. Warming up before doing anything athletic is not a new strategy, but warming up with the specific purpose of spiking your heart rate intermittently just prior to doing something that you know will give you anxiety is something very different. Here are some induced activities you can do to get that heart rate spiked. We acknowledge that your race venue may not permit you do some of them and in that case, some modification of the list below would also work.

"I think that everything is possible as long as you put your mind to it and you put the work and time into it. I think your mind really controls everything." - Michael Phelps

Self-Inducing Initial HR Spike

The intention of these exercises is to purposefully get you to be out of breath (T-level breathing).

1. If possible, jump in the water and do some very hard and fast strokes for no more than a few minutes. Take 10 strokes at maximum speed. Once out of breath, slow down briefly to catch your breath and then repeat.

2. Find an open space near the swim start and do some running suicide drills. These are very short and quick runs

back and forth for just a few minutes. Take a very short break between to lower your heart but quickly repeat.

3. Do some jumping jacks intervals. Very fast ones with arms and legs spread. Take a very short break between to lower your heart but quickly repeat.

During the brief break in these intervals, practice the breathing exercise with the intention of increasing your breathing counts (A-level breathing) to slow your heart rate. While doing so, recall both your skill and EQ focal thought for the swim. If you have to, mark these thoughts on your arm or wrist band so you can have a visual reminder during the swim.

Though you may still be nervous and anxious once this is done as you get started on the swim, you have tricked your body to lower levels of heart rate spikes, reducing the impact of the amygdala, and allowing you to access your memory for the all-important focal thoughts you need for your swim. You have essentially got the surprise of T-level breathing out of the way before the swim start, instead of in the first few hundred yards of the swim.

Once the swim has started, amidst the chaos, your first step is to use C-level breathing to find your EQ focal thought. Find that happy and perfect swim memory. This will further reduce your HR as the thought will be comforting, and you know this because you have used this swimming focal thought in training before and it worked. As soon as you have your EQ focal thought (perhaps it is the name of the venue of where you performed your best), then your mind is ready to find the complementary skill focal thought for your swim. It may be a pace stroke count or a body position. Whatever it is, get to it and you are ready to keep going, with both focal thoughts to guide you all the way in. These will allow you to remember to sight (your memory is not being held hostage), and use your YELLOW card ideas in the event that a mishap does occur. Obviously, you will not have your swim YELLOW card in the water, so you will need to repeat them over and over again until they are permanently etched in your memory. This can be done both as part of your pre-race checklist and during the intervals of self-induced HR spike.

"Setting a goal is not the only thing. It is deciding how you will go about achieving it and staying with the plan." - Tom Landry, former coach of the Dallas Cowboys

Go-to Stroke

Something you can work on is a go-to stroke. It is a swim stroke where the specific intention is to slow your HR. It is a minimalist stroke and done at a significantly slower pace. It can be breast stroke, side stroke, or whatever. It is something you have practiced and you know you can swim with this go-to stroke no matter what happens anywhere anytime for any length of time.

Practice Swimming with Others

It can be frightful if the first time that you get kicked or bumped around is on race-day. During training, a technique that can help you get comfortable being bumped around in the open water is to swim very close to 2 or 3 of your friends in the pool first and then in open water with the explicit intention of bumping each other, grabbing each other briefly, and having them try to knock your goggles out. This needs to be done with the intention of learning, not harming, so be careful and all parties must fully understand the intent of the practice! If these mishaps occur on race-day, then your brain will already have a memory of it and the threat factor (and subsequent anxiety spike) will be reduced. This is also the perfect time to concurrently practice your go-to stroke, breathing, and focal thoughts.

Hypoxic Swimming

A final technique worth exploring is hypoxic swimming. This is very similar to the self-induced anxiety spike. Swim 25 or 50 yards at full speed so that you are totally out of breath. Immediately after, proactively use your go-to stroke to lower your heart rate. Once your heart rate goes down (should not take you more than another 25 yards), repeat the exercise. This type of short practice can be invaluable during your race-day swim as you will likely experience similar highs and lows depending on when and where any mishaps occur. During the race-day swim if you have any mishap and your heart rate spikes, think of this go-to stroke and this hypoxic practice you have done to first lower your heart rate to access your EQ focal and subsequent skill focal thought.

Escape from Alcatraz Triathlon Swim: What an amazing race this is put on by Tri-California. The most unique and talked about part on the race is the swim. This is no easy swim when you have to take into consideration the distance, bitter cold water, and extremely strong currents. The first year I did this race I didn't fully understand how the currents worked although there was no shortage of advice and opinions flying my way from other athletes. Logically it was a giant mind game as the ferry took you out to Alcatraz for the start. You could see the transition in the distance which was northeast of the drop point. The challenge however was swimming in a northwest direction in order to get there. Needless to say having no chance to practice ahead of time I went way off course, completely underestimating the strength of the currents. As a result I ended up about 1,000 meters east of transition. I did not prepare enough mentally and logistically for this race.

Here is another example that I experienced of a swim mishap. The truth is many ocean swims can get rough and some athletes experience sea-sickness or nausea. It was my first time competing in the World Championships in Kona. Two days prior to the race, the water was really rough and I had my first experience with nausea. What I learned that day, and part of my solution for dealing with the challenge on race-day, was to (1) wear a patch, and (2) if I swallowed salt water, I knew that I would need to drink only water for the first 20 minutes on the ride and not to mix salty sea water with my EFS which could cause some GI issues. Water only would help clear anything from the sea and the nausea. Lesson, assess your situation and have a plan in mind for dealing with possible challenges.

-Heather Gollnick

Complete the exercises below to prepare for race-day swim.

Exercise: Your Potential Race-day Swim Mishaps

Make a list of 10 race-day swim mishaps that could happen to you. For each one, think of a solution. Then, during training, purposefully induce one or more of these mishaps and see if your solution would work.

1. Mishap:

   _____

   _____

   Solution: _____

   _____

   _____

2. Mishap:

   _____

   _____

   Solution: _____

   _____

   _____

3. Mishap:

   _____

   _____

   Solution: _____

   _____

   _____

4. Mishap:

_____

_____

Solution: _____

_____

_____

5. Mishap:

_____

_____

Solution: _____

_____

_____

6. Mishap:

_____

_____

Solution: _____

_____

_____

7. Mishap:

_____

_____

Solution: _____

_____

_____

8. Mishap: _____

_____

_____

Solution: _____

_____

_____

9. Mishap: _____

_____

_____

Solution: _____

_____

_____

10. Mishap: _____

_____

_____

Solution: _____

_____

Top 3 Ideas
I learned from this chapter

1.

2.

3.

3 Action Steps
I will take immediately to incorporate the above learning into my race-day swim strategy

1.

2.

3.

Chapter Summary

1. The swim start of a triathlon often times causes the greatest levels of anxiety in athletes.

2. It is your perception of threat that is at the heart of your anxiety.

3. Practice potential mishaps in training before they occur during a race. For every potential mishap, have a possible solution prepared in your mind to help alleviate elevated levels of anxiety.

Chapter 7
Race-Day Bike

From Linsey Corbin - Professional Triathlete

I try and put myself in situations during training so that on race-day, I am "comfortable with the uncomfortable." I try to experience challenging situations and times when I have to dig deep during big bike sessions (climbing a mountain pass or doing trainer intervals or a flat all-out time-trial) so that on race-day it is familiar territory. I often find that it is during the bike portion of an Ironman when I encounter those famous "high and low" points. When I reach a portion of the 112 mile bike where I start to struggle (this usually hits around mile 80), I go through a quick mental check list, starting with my nutrition: Have I eaten recently? How is my hydration? Have I taken salt tablets? Then I go through my body and sort of hit a re-set button: How is my cadence? Are my feet level with the pedal stroke? Am I relaxed through the hips? How is my posture? Is my head still? Lastly, I take a few deep breaths in and out to just simply, relax. Through experience I have learned that riding through the low points has its perks because they rarely last forever. It's just a matter of putting your head down, getting through it, and knowing that you will feel good in another few miles. I really embrace these challenges during the race!

Once out of the swim, you are on your way to the transition area (T1). And yes, all kinds of things can go wrong in T1 too. We recommend you perform a similar exercise as in the previous chapter with potential mishaps in T1. For the most part, they are few and, typically, there is enough support within the area to help you.

You are now on the bike. There are three sets of challenges you will face that will test your emotional strength as much as your physical ability. They are (i) pacing strategy, (ii) nutrition and hydration strategy, and (iii) an EQ strategy for those unpredictable mishaps.

"It isn't the mountains ahead to climb that wear you out; it's the pebble in your shoe." - Muhammad Ali

Potential Bike Mishaps

As we did in the previous chapter, it is worth making a list of all the mishaps that could potentially happen during your bike. Here are some common ones:

- Flat tire

- Losing water bottles

- Losing your nutrition packs

- Unexpected cross or head winds

- Duped into keeping pace with other bikers; abandoning your pacing strategy; inconsistency in your pacing

- Forgetting to eat and drink

- Hitting something on the road that misaligns your wheels

- Getting stung by a bee

- Rain making roads slippery

- Riding hills too hard

- Forgetting to be in aero position

- Penalty for drafting or blocking, or worse littering.

- Difficulties clipping in

- Inexplicable pain in some part of your body

- Dropping chain

- Experiencing a crash

- Making a wrong turn

- Bike computer stops working

Pacing Strategy

Once on the bike, you have now entered, from a purely racing perspective, the area where the race is won or lost. With the exception of sprint triathlons where the objective is to hammer all legs of the race as hard and fast as possible, in Olympic, half and full triathlons, your pacing on the bike will dictate how well you will be able to run and avoid bonking. Bike pacing is one of the more mentally challenging parts of a triathlon. It is challenging because riding *for* a run is very different from just riding. Many triathletes hit the bike a lot harder than they should which compromises their run pace. Triathletes that are often disappointed with their finish times almost always point to their slower run times not realizing that the potential cause of it was actually the bike pace. They will often say, "I had a terrible run, but my bike time was fantastic." Well, to be successful and optimize all your potential, you have to be good at all three legs and really focus on your bike pacing.

An analysis was done on two professional athletes competing in a full ironman distance. Both triathletes came out of the water at about the same time. The analysis specifically examined wattage (i.e., energy output for effort on the bike) of both riders who were chosen because they had similar targets of power to hit. One of the pros said that he quite unexpectedly had one of the best swims of his career and felt incredibly relaxed and energized when starting to bike. As a result, he decided he would ride about 10-20 watts more than his initial strategy. He was well ahead of his competitor until about mile 80 of the bike when he began to feel very fatigued. He eventually got caught and passed by the competitor and, in fact, did not finish the run.

If this can happen to professionals, it can and does happen to age-groupers all the time and is often noted as the biggest strategic mistake made by most triathletes. There appears to be either a high level of positive anxiety once out of the water to hit the bike hard, or a high level of impatience with sticking to a strategy that demands you go slower than what you are capable of on the bike.

This is an area where you can be at a significant advantage if you have a power meter on your bike as it directly measures your energy output. Based on your strategy, say 75% of your functional threshold power for a Half Ironman, you have a specific target to hit in order to run 13.1 miles after the bike at a run pace you have worked on and tested in calibration rides during training. Heart Rate (HR) zones can also be used, though not nearly as effective as power meters. Speed is not the best metric to use on your bike as it does not take into account energy you are exerting on hills, turns you may have to make, impact of wind, and other variables. With or without a power meter or HR monitor, we recommend you work specifically on figuring out the appropriate pace strategy for your bike leg.

Once you have a pacing strategy, then it is simply a matter of having the discipline of sticking to it, by not letting the emotions of the situation get to you the way it did for the pro in the example above. Here again is where taking your emotional temperature every 15 minutes (by setting an alarm on your watch or bike computer) can be very helpful. In addition, this is also the place where your macro focus, skill and EQ focal thoughts can be helpful to remind you to stick to your strategy. Use 'free-speed' areas (downhills, tail winds, etc.) to practice some A-level breathing.

Pacing comes down to managing your EQ. I see way too many athletes, even with power meters and heart rate monitors, ignore pacing in the heat of "competition". As an all too familiar example, if a woman passes a male competitor, some "ego button" must go off in males because more times than not, he will do everything in his power to pass her back. Even if he started in a wave prior to hers. This is a mistake I have witnessed with age-groupers so many times – they see that number on the back of a fellow competitor's leg and it's the same age group as theirs and wham – they try to hit that next gear. In the process they forsake their plan and target goals and often times blow up prior to hitting the finish line.

This mindset of competing against another athlete no matter what the circumstance often times happens in training as well. Recently I had an athlete doing a long ride in preparation for Ironman, working on nutrition, pacing, and holding a prescribed heart rate. He happened to be doing a great job but when a group of friends came by doing a much shorter, more intense ride, he not only joined in but ended up pulling the group. His heart rate was 20+ beats higher than prescribed and he expended too much energy going anaerobic which led to a rapid burning of his glycogen stores. He ended up bonking 15 miles later. The lesson here - stick to your pacing strategy!

-Heather Gollnick

Nutrition/Hydration Strategy

Your body is burning a lot of calories. On the bike, you are now depleting your body storage of glycogen and fueling becomes another key part of the race that can often be more of an emotional challenge than a physical one. It takes discipline, like in pacing, to consume what you need to at the time you need it. Your nutrition and hydration strategy comes from your training, is unique to you, and tied to your run strategy as well. Race-day is not the right day to test a new drink or food. Whatever you consume, test it extensively in your training (this can be a purpose itself for some of your workouts) before race-day. Different brands of the same product can potentially be very upsetting to your stomach so make sure you use on race-day exactly what you have been using in training.

It is easy to get lost in the moment and forget to consume the right amount of nutrition only to feel it later in the ride or most certainly in the run. By managing your monologues, having great macro focus to both be present and enjoy the moment, and by using your focal thoughts, you allow yourself the opportunity to execute your strategy and not to be impatient with yourself, especially when you are passed on the bike by others. Similar to the swim, the bike leg is a place where monologues will occur and this is where your advanced selection of positive and EQ-enabling monologues will be key.

Remember, for most of you, your bike leg is all about the set up for the run leg.

The following excerpt from a race report from an athlete I coach highlights the need for lessons learned, specifically as it relates to a good nutrition plan on the bike.

There were 30-40mph winds in our face along with a net gain of 3000 feet of altitude for the next 60 miles. At this point, I had a good feeling about my nutrition strategy. I had 5 sandwiches in a fanny pack and as an emergency I had 3 gels taped to my bike. I also had a concentrated bottle of EFS and 2 other water bottles, one being an aero bottle. I couldn't wait to try out my gourmet meal but my plan was to wait about an hour before my feast. Along the way I was sipping water, planning on about 1 bottle per hour with the EFS being diluted in my aero bottle.

After an hour on the bike, I had finished the water in the aero bottle and I was to squirt a little of the concentrated EFS into the aero bottle and dilute it with my other caged water bottle. I guess in the heat of the battle I forgot the EFS bottle was concentrated and I dumped all of the contents into the aero bottle. Now I'm in a predicament because I can't drink out of the aero bottle as the contents were too strong/concentrated. I can't dump the contents without un-strapping the aero bottle which would result in wasted time. As it turned out those precious minutes were meaningless, the race took me over 13 hours to complete. My solution was to sip the concentrated EFS out of the bottle and spit it out until the level was low enough to add water for dilution. There goes my liquid nutrition unless I use the Ironman Perform at the aid stations which I dislike. However, I do have my sandwiches! That leads me to the next problem. I started eating my highly anticipated meal and it didn't taste the way I had envisioned. I like all the ingredients but when they are in that combination, yuck. I guess I won't have my own cooking show on the gourmet network. I should have done a trial run with this combination beforehand which was strongly suggested by my coach. For the next four hours I was only able to tolerate a total of two sandwiches, the rest I threw away.

So here I am at the 6 1/2 hour mark having consumed only 2 gels, 2 sandwiches, 1 bottle of EFS as my only nutrition and it is starting to feel like it. I was a little concerned about how my nutrition strategy was going. At my current rate of speed, or lack of, I calculated my time on the bike was going to last another 1 1/2 hours. That's when I started eyeing my emergency ration of 3 gels. I never really liked gels that much, that is why I opted for the sandwich routine. I took a gel and started feeling better almost immediately, psychosomatic? Maybe, nevertheless, it was working. However, I had already dug myself a hole nutritionally which was to play a factor for the rest of the race. For the remaining bike segment my pace was slowing. I was able to force down some Ironman Perform and a few banana slices along with the remaining two gels I had on board. I didn't take the gels that were offered at the aid stations because I still didn't like the taste. I was able to keep my legs moving to get to the next phase....the marathon.

Starting the marathon was anticlimactic. All my lofty goals I had set for myself had disintegrated on the bike and I just wanted to finish. During the run I hooked up with another competitor and we pushed each other until we crossed the finish line in just over 13 hours. It was almost surreal to finish my first Ironman even though my time was disappointing to me.

However, I took home some important lessons that I would apply to my next race. Listen to your coach. I had a 5-Time Ironman Champion helping me with training and nutrition strategies and I didn't take advantage of her knowledge. I thought I knew better.

As it turned out, I followed Heather's plan on my next race and I went from a disappointing finish in St George to qualifying for Kona in NYC by coming in 3rd in my age group!

-Heather Gollnick

EQ Strategy

Compared to Norman Stadler discussed earlier, in 2011 Chrissie Wellington (who was also the defending World Triathlon Champion) was once again building a large lead on the bike at Kona when she experienced a flat tire. Chrissie replaced the tire but pulled the CO2 cartridge too early and had no air to pump up her tire. She stood on the roadside helpless asking her fellow competitors for a spare cartridge. Unlike Stadler, Chrissie didn't panic. It took about 10 minutes for her to finally get a cartridge and was quickly back on the Queen "K" working her way back into the lead. She then set a record with a great marathon run and claimed her second straight title.

I actually had a sticker of a stop light on my bike for an entire season. It served as a reminder that despite all the things that can go wrong on the bike, my emotional response was key. It was ok to go from green to yellow but with controlled emotions the quicker you got back to green the more ideal (and not getting to red). I teach my athletes the importance of remembering to train your mind to go from yellow back to green in a race without falling to red, thereby guaranteeing, in large measure, a successful race outcome. Developing these kind of mental strategies has been a key to my success – in over 250 race starts, I have only DNF'd twice due to injury. You must recognize that if not managed correctly, your emotions can spiral you out of control.

-Heather Gollnick

Bike Mechanics

"When the spirits are low, when the day appears dark, when work becomes monotonous, when hope hardly seems worth having, just mount a bicycle and go out for a spin down the road, without thought on anything but the ride you are taking." - Arthur Conan Doyle

An effective strategy on the bike is not just about a good pacing strategy, a good hydration/nutrition strategy, and a good EQ strategy. It is also about having some basic knowledge about your equipment, the bike, and having tools to fix things. As triathletes, you should know how to inflate your tires, change a flat, fix a dropped chain, adjust break-pads, etc. For example, understanding how to change a flat is something you must learn to do. And you should practice this several times before your race. Even if you know how to change a tire, you must also learn the nuance of a CO_2 cartridge which, as described earlier, even a world champion can mess up on. Go to your bike shop or take several clinics on bike maintenance and repair. You never know, these skills might make all the difference on race–day!

Refuel Your EQ Tank

Your glycogen is not the only thing being depleted as the race progresses. Unlike the swim, on the bike your five senses are exposed to much more stimuli that can be used to your advantage. You are on roads passing cheering fans, volunteers at aid stations and turns, neighborhoods, beaches, mountains, and all the sounds and smells that come with them. Each one can be a powerful refueling stimulus for your emotional energy that you have rapidly depleting as you work to stay focused for hours. As your body begins to fatigue after hours of swimming and biking, and your brain begins to divert attention to your aching legs and other sore body parts, you are also depleting your EQ that you need for all the focus, focal thoughts, and positive monologues.

One athlete we work with had an EQ Focal Thought of saying "thank you" a hundred times on the bike to volunteers and fans and two hundred times on the run. She counted every time she did it. She made sure that when she said thank you, she also smiled. This is not something she could do on the swim, but she fully executed this EQ refueling strategy in addition to her overall EQ strategy and was one of the few people to finish with a huge smile on her face. Her positive attitude, she contended afterwards, was the glue for her in all the hours and minutes at the different points in the race to stick to GREEN. She said she never got to RED on her EQ temperature all day despite a couple of mishaps and it was much easier to recall her YELLOW cards and other EQ plans during those mishaps in much the same way Chrissie Wellington kept her calm during her flat tire.

Complete the exercises below to prepare for your race-day bike.

Exercise: Your Potential Race-day Bike Mishaps

Make a list of 10 race-day bike mishaps that could happen to you. For each one, think of a solution. Then, during training, purposefully induce one or more of these mishaps and see if your solution would work.

1. Mishap: _____

_____

Solution: _____

_____

_____

2. Mishap: _____

_____

Solution: _____

_____

_____

3. Mishap: _____

_____

Solution: _____

_____

_____

4. Mishap:

    _____

    _____

    Solution: _____

    _____

    _____

5. Mishap:

    _____

    _____

    Solution: _____

    _____

    _____

6. Mishap:

    _____

    _____

    Solution: _____

    _____

    _____

7. Mishap:

    _____

    _____

Solution: _____

_____

_____

8. Mishap:

_____

_____

Solution: _____

_____

_____

9. Mishap:

_____

_____

Solution: _____

_____

_____

10. Mishap:

_____

_____

Solution: _____

_____

Top 3 Ideas
I learned from this chapter

1.

2.

3.

3 Action Steps
I will take immediately to incorporate the above
learning into my race-day bike strategy

1.

2.

3.

Chapter Summary

1. Your race-day pacing strategy, nutrition plan, and EQ strategy are key elements to a well-executed bike leg.

2. Practice your pacing strategy, nutrition plan, and EQ preparation throughout your training before race-day.

3. Practice potential bike mishaps in training before they occur during a race. For every potential mishap, have a solution prepared.

Chapter 8
Race-Day Run

From Meredith Kessler - 4 Time Ironman Champion

I passed out at Ironman St. George on mile twenty-two of the run two years ago while I was in 2nd place due to an imbalance of sodium and electrolytes. Six weeks later at Ironman Coeur D'Alene, a similar situation happened due to too much sodium during the race where my kidneys were unable to process the sodium causing massive water weight gain and disorientation which resulted in another DNF back to back. I never wanted to feel this way again so I did extensive research to figure out what went wrong. I eliminated the culprit of sodium citrate, increased my electrolyte consumption, and drank more liquids before and during the race. The worry of passing out again pushed me to correct the problems and I am always cognizant of not repeating the mistakes of the past for this very reason. The key to success is staying calm, being willing to troubleshoot, and finding innovative ways to overcome the obstacles at hand.

You have successfully completed the bike and back in the transition area (T2). T2 typically tends to be easier as it involves dismounting from your bike, finding your transition area, getting your run shoes on, race belt, hat, and off you go. Mishaps can happen in T2 also, and so it is incumbent on you to prepare yourself for them. Just as in the previous chapter in T1, you may wish to make a list of potential mishaps in T2 and how you would address them.

The professionals will tell you that the run is where the race really begins. The common adage of 'swim for warm up, bike for show, run for dough' certainly applies.

As with the bike, there are three sets of challenges you will face that will test your emotional strength as much as your physical ability. They are (i) pacing strategy, (ii) nutrition and hydration strategy, and (iii) EQ strategy. The EQ strategy during the run is not just for those unpredictable mishaps, but more so for the fact that your body will physically be at the most stressed level of the race, and where your monologues will sound like screaming matches. The run is where you will need to muster all your EQ training.

> When I race and have a physical or emotional hurdle and I'm not sure if I have the effort to overcome it, I try to think ahead about how I will feel the day after the race or even two days later if I don't give it 100% that day, both physically and mentally. Pushing yourself hard can mean dealing with pain or discomfort physically, but in comparison, the emotional pain of disappointment of not pushing myself through race day trials is much harder to swallow, particularly as a professional.
>
> *-Heather Gollnick*

Potential Run Mishaps

As we did in the previous chapter, it is worth making a list of all the mishaps that could potentially happen during your run. Here are some common ones:

- Intense fatigue

- Sudden inexplicable pain

- Taking a wrong turn

- Getting stung by a bee

- Blisters

- Indigestion

- Feeling sunburn

- Heavy shoes from rain

- Weather changes requiring hydration strategy change

- Shoelaces keep loosening

- Forget to eat/drink

- Your wrist watch computer stops working

Pacing Strategy

Depending on the distance of your triathlon and the venue conditions, your run strategy may change. There are run routes where a single loop is used, or where multiple loops are used, and others where it is point to point.

The nature of your run route may dictate your run strategy. For example, in a popular Olympic distance triathlon in the Appalachian Mountains, the 10K is an out and back. The first 5K is a very steep climb, followed by a fairly rapid decent back for the other 5K. This is not a route where you can afford to hit it hard going uphill assuming that gravity will somehow pull you down the hill – you still have to run down which, if not done carefully, can lead to injury. This run route dictates a very different type of hill training to get your legs accustomed to both the up and down hill run. In addition, it requires a totally different running technique and pacing strategy up the hill, then down the hill. Our main point here is that you should study your run route and its geography (elevation, shade, terrain) so that when you are experiencing it during race-day your brain is not surprised and sending off threat alerts at a time when you are at your highest level of fatigue.

In addition to the route and terrain, there is also a pacing strategy. This is something you will need to work on during your training. It is not unusual to break the run into different phases which mentally are more manageable. The most commonly used one is a negative split where you run the first half a little conservatively and the second half much more aggressively. This works particularly well for shorter distances like a sprint or Olympic.

At the half and full ironman distances, the pacing strategy may be different. For example, a common one for the half is to break the 13.1 miles into three segments. Athletes will use the first 3 miles as a warm up, slower in pace to get your body accustomed to transitioning from being on the bike to running. The next 7 miles are at your target pace, and then, depending on how your body is doing, to be much more aggressive the last 3 miles towards the finish. A full ironman distance might use a similar break up but perhaps have four segments.

You can see how having a plan to execute can be invaluable during the run as it is something you know will work for you based on your training. Your run pacing strategy, based on your bike effort, is one of the most important items to determine during training.

Nutrition/Hydration Strategy

When you eat something, visualize it giving you energy. I know that glycogens give me energy. I know that nutrition is a tough part in an ironman tri. When I fuel, I mentally feel the food and energy coming into my system giving me the energy that I need. My muscles are fatigued but when I eat a waffle or gel, I visualize how it is fueling my muscles. Oh, I feel the boost! The mind is a powerful tool.

-Heather Gollnick

Your body is well past its own storage of glycogen (fuel) and if you have been doing a good job of nutrition/hydration on the bike, then it is only a matter of continuing to do so for the run. The key term here is 'continuing to do so.'

Just like the bike, it takes discipline to consume what you need during the run at the time you need to. Your nutrition and hydration strategy comes from your training, is unique to you, and tied to your run strategy as well.

It is easy to get lost in the moment and forget to fuel, only to feel it later in the run. Similar to the bike leg, there are typically aid stations every couple of miles or so during the run leg. These stations are full of different kinds of drinks and food. While race-day is not the right day to test a new drink or food, venues will often announce in advance what kind of fuel and at which miles aid stations will be offered. Whatever you consume, test it extensively in your training (this can be a purpose itself for some of your workouts) before race-day. Different brands of the same product can potentially be very upsetting to your stomach so make sure you use on race-day exactly what you have been using in training.

EQ Strategy

Ask people "what do you say to yourself when you look in the mirror?" They may say, "I need to shave" or "OMG my wrinkles" or "Where is all my hair?" or "I was so slow today"! Think of all those negative things we do and say when we look in the mirror. How many times do you say, "I look good?" or "Love my smile" or "World, here I come!" or "Way to get up and train today." What we say to ourselves can affect our whole day and frame of mind.

-Heather Gollnick

"I run because long after my footprints fade away, maybe I will have inspired a few to reject the easy path, hit the trails, put one foot in front of the other, and come to the same conclusion I did: I run because it always takes me where I want to go." - Dean Karnazes

Although most accidents occur in the swim and bike legs of the race, it is the run portion that requires the most out of your EQ strategy. Even though you've been fueling properly throughout your race, your body is also heavily fatigued and being filled with new chemicals (hormones) whose specific instinctive purpose is to convince you to slow down and give up (in order to preserve your body from any amount of pain). Remember, the primary purpose of any living creature is self-preservation. Our DNA is built to do so. In order for your body to give up, it has to gets its orders from the brain. So the brain is going to its most established memories (negative ones) and neuro-pathways (ways of thinking). These come in conflict with your training and your desire to succeed. Monologues quickly turn to internal dialogues with negative and positive thoughts taking turns to convince you to give up or keep going. These battles can easily derail you from following your pacing and nutrition/hydration strategy. Often times, by the time the battling monologues take a break, you are well past a distance where you had intended to eat, drink, or check your pacing.

The run is the perfect opportunity to take everything you have learned in this book and put it into action. You understand how the brain works and how emotions dictate the chemical composition of your body and ability to physically perform.

We will outline here a specific EQ run strategy for a half ironman distance race. For your specific distance, you will have to modify this plan to meet your distances.

Graphically, irrespective of your race distance, break your run into three distinct phases knowing that the first phase, miles 0-3, you will be likely be in GREEN mode. As you begin to fatigue and get into the teeth of the run, miles 3-10, you will likely be in YELLOW mode. As you approach the last phase, miles 10-13, you will be in RED mode. Because you can expect to be in these states, you already have cards to help you deal with each one to get you back to GREEN as often as possible.

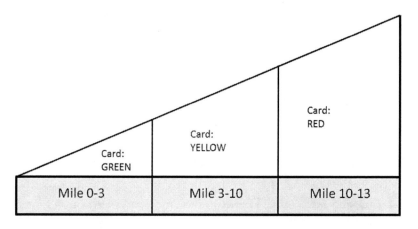

Figure 14. Run EQ Strategy

To be more specific, see the action items listed below for each phase.

Distance (mile)	EQ Action Item
0 – 3	Have your list of selected positive monologues playlist ready either on a card or written on your race belt or clothing. Focus on A-level breathing (slower counts in and out) and macro focus with your 5 senses. Incorporate run Skill and EQ Focal thoughts. Use Aid Stations points to trigger incorporating micro focus for just a minute or two after each station.

Take your EQ temperature every mile. Use an alarm feature on your watch to trigger this action. Pay close attention to the quality of your internal conversations; their tone, content, and speed. Listen to yourself as though you are eavesdropping on two people talking. If temperature is YELLOW, begin use of selected monologues and YELLOW Card content. Use the fans and volunteers as targets to smile at (or say "thank you") to help you stay in GREEN.

Distance (mile)	EQ Action Item
3 - 10	Once in positive monologue mode, focus exclusively on the Skill and EQ focal run thoughts. Slowly incorporate macro focus again. Use all your senses to notice everything around you. Fill up your EQ tank with positive memories and monologues. Your level of breathing should be at C level.
10 – 13	Unless there is a mishap of any kind (in which case you have your YELLOW and RED cards to help you get back to GREEN), stick with Skill Focal Thought but switch EQ focus to breathing (slower) and micro focus all the way in. Allow yourself to go back and forth between C- and T- level breathing while maintaining your desired pace.

You must believe that a triathlon is as much a test of your physical abilities as it is your emotional strength. Both are being tested and at no greater point than the run portion of your race. Remember, the run was all set up by an effective bike strategy that incorporated its own pacing, nutrition/hydration, and EQ strategies. The EQ Run Strategy we have outlined here should give you a great starting point to build your own plan for your race and distance.

A friend was preparing to run a marathon, and struggling just to get her mind around what she would think about for 26 miles. I had her make a list of 26 people and dedicate each mile to each person on that list, with the closest family members at the end. With each mile she thought about another important person in her life, and afterwards she thought the marathon went by so fast.

-Heather Gollnick

Take a look at your story in Chapter 1 where you underperformed. Could a bike strategy and a subsequent EQ-based run strategy have helped you?

Exercise: Your Run EQ Plan

Based on your next race, and the distance, **create your own run EQ Plan** here using the example provided earlier.

Distance (mile)	EQ Action Step
_____	_____
_____	_____
_____	_____
_____	_____
_____	_____
_____	_____
_____	_____
_____	_____
_____	_____

Write a Screenplay of Your Race

Two months before your race, write a script of how you want your race-day to go, both logistically and with an EQ strategy. What will you do the week of taper, physically and with EQ? Where will you stay? When to wake up? What to eat? What will you do all the way through to swim start? What do you want to be thinking about? How will you handle potential race-day mishaps? Address all scenarios that could happen in the script.

Read this script the week of taper before race-day as part of your EQ strategy for taper week. Reading it allows you to be in command of reaching your goals instead of leaving it up to random events and circumstances. For example, if you drop your water bottle, your script will remind you to turn around and get it. On race-day you do not have time to think about things like this. By reading your script, you already know how you would react.

> My first sports psychologist, Marc Strickland, had me write three types of goals; (A) Outcome, (B) Performance, & (C) Process. I find this exercise very important as the outcome goals are only part of the story. "How do you want to finish?" i.e., your outcome is a different question from "how do you want to "perform?" The performance is the process of getting to the outcome. Performance is more important and will lead to victory or PRs. I can have the best finish and win the race but not execute well, or I can do everything right and come in fifth. Which was a better race?
>
> *-Heather Gollnick*

Race-Day Goals

Complete the exercises below for your next race-day goals:

Exercise: Outcome Goal

When all is said and done I would like to:

_____

_____

_____

_____

Exercise: Performance Goals

These goals are restricted to specific behaviors such as "complete my swim in 1 hour." Developing these goals allows you control over your performance and the ability to appropriately evaluate the Performance. Focusing then on the performance gives you the best chance for success.

SWIM: _____

_____

BIKE: _____

_____

RUN: _____

_____

Exercise: Process Goals

How will you accomplish the above Performance Goals?

SWIM: _____

_____

BIKE: _____

_____

RUN: _____

_____

Write the Script

Based on your goals, write your race-day script. From the moment you wake up, until you cross the finish line, script out your day. Include everything. *I will wake up at….. I will eat …… for breakfast, I will feel…… , I will get to transition and ……., my swim strategy is…….., when I feel like things are getting tough this is what I will do, etc.…* Try to go through every detail of your day and script out your experience, then refer to it daily and build in that positive feeling: you are on your way to a great day.

Have in here a RED card entry that you know will have the same emotional impact as the daughter and mother-in-law in wheel chairs had on Heather Gollnick as she was literally on the verge of giving up on the run, only to go on and win the race (see Chapter 2 for Heather's story).

Exercise: Your Potential Race-day Run Mishaps

Make a list of 10 race-day run mishaps that could happen to you. For each one, think of a solution. Then, during training, purposefully induce one or more of these mishaps and see if your solution would work.

1. Mishap: _____

   _____

   Solution: _____

   _____

   _____

2. Mishap: _____

   _____

   Solution: _____

   _____

   _____

3. Mishap: _____

   _____

   Solution: _____

   _____

   _____

4. Mishap:

_____

_____

Solution: _____

_____

_____

5. Mishap:

_____

_____

Solution: _____

_____

_____

6. Mishap:

_____

_____

Solution: _____

_____

_____

7. Mishap:

_____

_____

Solution: _____

_____

_____

8. Mishap: _____

_____

Solution: _____

_____

_____

9. Mishap: _____

_____

Solution: _____

_____

_____

10. Mishap: _____

_____

Solution: _____

_____

Top 3 Ideas
I learned from this chapter

1.

2.

3.

3 Action Steps
I will take immediately to incorporate the above
learning into my race-day run strategy

1.

2.

3.

Chapter Summary

1. You must believe that a triathlon is as much a test of your physical abilities as it is your emotional strength (EQ), and the run is where you will be tested for this.

2. Your run EQ strategy should be broken into 3 phases, each having its own pre-planned EQ action items.

3. A race-day script, including logistics, EQ strategy, and process/outcome goals will better prepare you for the race.

Chapter 9
Recovery

From Ben Greenfield - Fitness Expert

Both my training and racing are subpar when I'm stressed. After a day of work, if I don't take a moment to pause and de-stress, my training suffers. Similarly, if I wake up on the morning of a race and go check e-mail or turn on my phone, it can also spell disaster. So I try and keep as stress-free as possible, especially during important training or racing weeks. One really useful stress-control method I employ is called "Heart Rate Variability" (HRV). I track my HRV every morning, and if it's too low, I do biofeedback exercises such as deep breathing and focusing on positive aspects of my life for which I'm grateful. If I can't get it to come down, then I know I'm not just mentally stressed, but I'm also physically smoked, so I take a full rest day - and that helps tremendously.

We have covered a great deal so far in this book. We have exposed you to emotional intelligence (EQ), the physiology of the body and brain, learning models, how to make your training more effective, and finally, applying all these concepts to your race-day disciplines of swim, bike, and run.

There are two more dimensions that we feel are important to address to help you get the most out of your body, and both have their basis in EQ. In this chapter, we will discuss one of them: Recovery. In the next chapter, we will discuss the other component: Life Balance.

Consider again the demographics and it is safe to assume that most of you are in your 30s and 40s. From a physiology perspective, this means that you do not have a young body that can recover from hard workouts nearly as well as you were able to a few years ago. But recovery is a critical part of training not just for older athletes, but also for everyone as the intensity of workouts takes a toll on all bodies. Over-training and incorrect training are an all too common phenomenon that work against triathletes.

"The man who views the world at 50 the same as he did at 20 has wasted 30 years of his life." - Muhammad Ali

Psychology of Training and Recovery

Physical training is an incredibly rewarding experience. According to the Mayo Clinic, working out helps combat health issues and diseases, manage weight, impact mood, boost energy, and promotes better sleep. For athletes, there are more reasons.

For me, working out is and always has been a mental and stress reliever. For example, when my newborn twins were in the hospital, I would run or walk around the block outside the hospital. After finally making it home with them after several months in the hospital, my mother-in-law would periodically come over for a few hours a week to help. I would say, "I'm so exhausted – I need to go out for a run!" Not being a runner that sounded very strange to her. "Why not take a nap?" she would ask. I knew if I went to lie down all I would do is think about our circumstances. Instead I would go for a run to clear my mind and experience a very necessary release from our stress.

-Heather Gollnick

For others, the competitive nature with peers is a big factor. Bragging rights till the next race are worth serious emotional capital.

Exercise: Reasons for Training
What are your true reasons for training?
1.
2.
3.

4.	
5.	

For triathletes, working out is an integral part of the routine of life. Not working out is actually more of an issue than working out itself. We hear triathletes all the time talking about missing a workout as though they were missing a very important business meeting or family commitment. They typically feel very guilty about missing a workout. Incorporating recovery for those athletes that work full-time and have a busy social life or a family is a very real challenge. It is understandable how athletes stretched for time would put recovery on the back burner to make sure they fit in every training opportunity possible.

> This area has always been the hardest area for me. As a professional triathlete, business owner and mother of three, I would always push recovery off. Having serious race ambitions and goals, I have often ignored minor injuries and raced anyway, only to have something minor turn into something major because I didn't listen to my body. I listened too much to that competitive voice in my head. Even now I have to constantly remind myself how essential recovery is. Over the years I have gotten better at this but I get it - recovery is tough!
>
> *-Heather Gollnick*

The psychology behind this guilt is something you should really try to understand. A very good question to ask is 'what impact does missing a workout truly have on your fitness or preparation for a race?' In most cases, the truthful answer is none. So why then is it so bothersome to so many?

Exercise: Missing Workouts
Why does it really bother you when you miss workouts?
1.
2.
3.
4.
5.

A set of more important questions to ask is why recovery is not given the same consideration as working out itself. One answer is that recovery does not result in fatigue and sweat (two feel-good outcomes of working out) and, therefore, we assume it is of no benefit. Related to this is the lack of the endorphin high you experience during workouts that you do not experience in recovery that may hinder you from fully recovering. In addition, most of us think of recovery as just a day off, and this is far from what we are talking about. Off days, considered as rest days, are in fact off days, as you saw in the sample training plan in Chapter 4. These rest days are critical for your body and for an effective preparation. Recovery is not just an off day as we will discuss in this chapter.

We love the commitment triathletes have to their fitness and preparation for a race and by no means want to dissuade you from continuing to do so. What we want to encourage you to do is to think of recovery as an integral part of your training.

Advantages of Recovery

1. Allow for body to recover from hard workouts

2. Allow body to prepare for future hard workouts

3. Better sleep

4. Prevent injury

5. Reduce emotional stress (allowing for refilling of EQ Tank)

6. Removal of metabolic waste

7. Prevent burn out

8. Restore balance and reduce overload

Note that none of the above can occur if you are training hard all the time.

"Run and become. Become and run. Run to succeed in the outer world. Become to proceed in the inner world." - Sri Chinmoy

Active Recovery

Active recovery is a wonderful way to incorporate the benefits of recovery while still being active. You are still working out but doing so at a very low intensity. Active recovery is strongly recommended in between hard workouts such as long runs or rides. Examples of active recovery are listed below, but keep in mind that a measure of active recovery is your ability to be mostly at A-level breathing:

- Low intensity swim

- Short HR Zone 1 run or bike

- Yoga or Pilates

- Core or stretch workout

- Massage

- Midday power naps

- Mastering EQ by practicing 3:1 EQ Ratio Principle by visualization

- Walk

- Ice Bath

- Filling up your EQ Tank (practice for taper week)

By reviewing this list, you can see how the paradigm of recovery being just an off-day begins to shift. Some of you may have to embed some or all of these into your training plan. Doing so takes an emotional competence and satisfaction.

There are also days when you wake up and just do not have it. Perhaps you have a nagging injury or just not in the right mood for a long hard workout. Listening to your body by taking your emotional temperature and realizing you are not in GREEN is key to a productive workout. A healthy compromise with yourself might be to do an active recovery workout.

Sleep

Sleep is another key part of recovery. Studies indicate that an average athlete needs about 8-9 hours of sleep a day. Consider that most triathletes work out in the mornings before going to work or juggling other family commitments, it is common to cut into this required sleep time for the workout. If this resonates with you, then mastering the skill of sleeping itself is a key competency for you as a triathlete. Again, it will require emotional competence, not physical, to orchestrate a sleep strategy.

Professional triathletes are notoriously protective of their sleep. When traveling, many are known to take their own beds, pillows, and other personalized sleep essentials with them on the road. They have also figured out a go-to-sleep routine that works for them. For many, it means going to bed earlier, cutting off all electronics several hours before intended sleep time to avoid keeping-me-awake thoughts. It also means not having any caffeine, sugars or any other type of food that will compromise their sleep. We also encourage athletes to take their EQ temperature as they begin their sleep routine and use the YELLOW card in the same manner as in competition to address any negative monologues so that they can be substituted with positive ones that would allow you to sleep.

> Adequate sleep can be a challenge for anyone, particularly athletes. Many times I have gone to bed knowing that I need to get 8 hours of sleep because I understand how important it is for my recovery. If I didn't fall asleep right away, I used to look at my watch and say, ok if I fall asleep now then I will get 7.5 hours, then that suddenly turns into 7 hours then down to six. I've learned not to put needless pressure on myself, take deep breaths, and try to let my sleep come naturally.
>
> *-Heather Gollnick*

As triathletes, you are encouraged to measure your sleep during your triathlon season and embrace a sleep routine much like the professionals do.

Sleep and active recovery are also essential to your EQ. There is a finite amount of emotional energy you have each day and it needs to be spread around all of life's activities, not just your hard workouts. Recovery and active recovery are both excellent times to refuel your EQ tank.

As a coach, I build it into training plans and it seems to take the guilt away. I now find myself putting recovery workouts into my own plan and I have learned to enjoy the easy 30 minute spin and stretch days. These lessons aren't easy to learn but they are necessary. For instance, in 2007, I had just won an Ironman and was excited to compete in what would be my fourth Ironman that season soon after that victory. The season before I had competed in 3 and finished in the top 3 in all events. "Why not four?" I asked myself, I was on another roll. The answer for me was Adrenal Fatigue (Adrenal fatigue is a collection of signs and symptoms that results when the adrenal glands function below the necessary level - the symptom is fatigue that is not relieved by sleep). Despite the symptoms I kept pushing myself both mentally and physically. My goals were too important and I couldn't stop despite my growing level of fatigue. It wasn't until I was told what I was experiencing that I slowed down and allowed my body to recover.

-Heather Gollnick

"Sleep is the best meditation." - Dalai Lama

Pete Jacobs Principle

The 2012 Kona World Champion has a wonderful way of thinking about recovery. As a professional athlete who has the time to train all day and every day, he confessed it was hard for him at first to embrace recovery activities. He then decided that his goal for each day would be to have several workouts and to count recovery workouts as part of his quota for the day. He gave an example of taking an afternoon nap as one of the quotas for the day. As long as he met his quota for the day, it did not matter what he did and he'd start to both feel better about recovery, and also see improvements in his workouts and performance.

So you, too, are encouraged to think of your recovery workouts as part of your weekly quota of workouts and we are certain you will see the same results as Pete did.

"I am building a fire, and every day I train, I add more fuel. At just the right moment, I light the match." - Mia Hamm

Build Your Recovery Plan

Exercise: Activities For Immediate Integration
From the list of active recovery activities we have listed, pick 5 that you feel you can integrate immediately into your training plan.
1.
2.
3.
4.
5.

Exercise: Current Sleep Routine

Write down your current go-to-sleep routine, if you have one

Exercise: Sleep Routine Modifications

Write down modifications to your sleep routine so that you can ensure 8-9 hours of quality sleep

---

Top 3 Ideas
I learned from this chapter

1.

2.

3.

3 Action Steps
I will take immediately to incorporate
recovery into my training plan

1.

2.

3.

Chapter Summary

1. For triathletes, working out is an integral part of the routine of life. Not working out is actually more of an issue than working out itself.

2. Recovery needs to be given the same amount of consideration as working out.

3. Think of your recovery workouts as part of your weekly quota of workouts.

Chapter 10
Life Balance

Excerpt from Chris "Macca" McCormack – January, 2013, issue of TRIATHLETE

Kona 2012 didn't go as planned. On race-day I was empty, and the event was over before it began. I sat confused and flat in my house after the race. My kids were running around laughing and screaming, tanned from a day in the sun. As I sat there trying to work out what went wrong, what mistakes we could have made in the preparation, what had left me so weak and soft in the race, I tried to laugh and just be normal for them.

My eldest daughter, Tahlia, sat down next to me, threw her arms around me, and in her soft, innocent voice said, "Dad, don't be sad!"

I looked at her and smiled, realizing I had been lost in a chasm of my thoughts. "Darling, Dad is not sad! I am just disappointed. That's all! I can be better, and that makes Dad disappointed!"

Tahlia looked at me a little confused and then said with some purpose, "Well, Dad, maybe that was your today best! That doesn't

179

mean your tomorrow best can't be better than your today best! Be the best you can be today, Dad. And then tomorrow be the best you can be tomorrow. When you do that, you will be the best dad you can be, and that's the most important thing."

I was shocked! She absolutely floored me. When did my 8-year-old get so philosophical? I looked at her so proudly, shaking my head in a moment of realization and disbelief.

In the preceding chapter, we said that there were two additional dimensions to successful performance with recovery being the first. The second one is the Balance of Life.

Referencing again to the demographics of you, the triathlete, it is safe to assume that you are in an adult relationship, have children, and a good job. This means you are responsible for all the things that come with being a father, mother, significant other, neighbor, friend, brother, sister, uncle, aunt, relative, co-worker, boss, and the like. You may also have relationships with non-profits, religious or spiritual organizations, and other clubs with other activities that you enjoyed before you got into triathlons.

Dozens of workplace studies from as far back as the 1960s have shown that "happy" workers are actually more productive than "unhappy" workers. Happy workers tended to get more done in the same amount of time than unhappy workers. Hopefully there is no argument against what might seem obvious in these findings. Having worked with dozens of athletes in all sports, we have found the same to be true for all athletes. Happy athletes tend to be more focused, be able to find focus when it is not there, and perform more consistently at higher levels than those that are not happy.

"Just as your car runs more smoothly and requires less energy to go faster and farther when the wheels are in perfect alignment, you perform better when your thoughts, feelings, emotions, goals, and values are in balance." - Brian Tracy

Now, you may start to feel uncomfortable wondering why a book on triathlons is talking about happiness in the last chapter. Our response is simple – a happy triathlete will perform close to their potential better than an unhappy one. Using the concepts of this book, a happy triathlete is in GREEN both in and out of training and races. It is very difficult to be YELLOW or RED in your personal life and then forcibly switch to GREEN during training or when you need to most, during a race.

> Years ago, I coached a successful traveling business man training for an Ironman. He was obsessed with training. As soon as he got back in town, his first stop was the gym. In addition, the weekends were spent working out, again away from home and his family. He was missing Little League games, and spending time with his kids and his wife was becoming a real challenge. His inability to find the right balance had made those important to him unhappy, and as a result, made him unhappy too. His workouts became more aggressive and lacked focus. His performance suffered. He got injured because he kept pushing, and finally got sidelined. During his recovery, he was the happiest he had been in years because he finally took the time to give his loved ones the attention they needed and deserved.
>
> *-Heather Gollnick*

The purpose of this chapter is to help you analyze your life so that you can have balance, and happiness, as a result. This has a direct impact on performance and that is why we are writing this chapter. There are several important exercises in this chapter that we ask you to take as seriously as all the other exercises we have asked you to do in the previous chapters.

"Sports do not build character. They reveal it." - Heywood Broun

Know what needs to be balanced

The first step in having a balance is to know what exactly it is that needs balancing. We assumed in the example above that it was spouse and kids, but this may not be true for some of you. Knowing what needs to be balanced will in turn make it clear for you to balance them.

Who are you?

No, this is not a philosophical question. In fact, it is a very pragmatic question. Each one of us plays many roles in our lives.

Exercise: Your Ten Most Important Roles
In no prioritized order, please list the ten most important roles to you:
1.
2.
3.
4.

5.	
6.	
7.	
8.	
9.	
10.	

Your Circle of Life

In the chart below, and from the list above, take the top five most important roles you need to play in the next 12 months, and insert them into the circles around you.

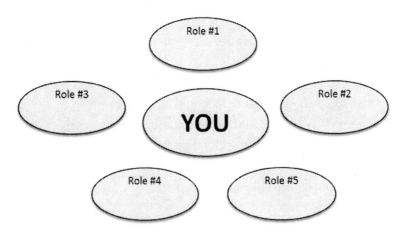

This represents your EQ universe. These roles are so important to you, that your performance in ALL of them will dictate your performance in EACH one of them.

"Sports are a microcosm of society." - Billie Jean King

Monitor Your EQ Day

Up until now we have asked you to center your EQ strategy on training and race-day. We have taught you how to transition from work or home life into triathlete life so that you can be focused with the purpose of your training (Chapter 5). We have also shown you how to do the same for race-day and during each leg of the triathlon. But according to your EQ Universe above, your being a triathlete is only one part of your world, one fifth of your EQ tank. Daily or weekly, as you enter the other roles in your universe, roles that collectively will determine your happiness (GREEN state), you will need to execute the same EQ strategy described in previous chapters of measuring your EQ temperature and using the tools we have given you to make sure that before entering the other roles, you are in GREEN mode. Though these other roles are different in terms of logistics, time, and skill requirement, they are identical in their EQ requirement of you being GREEN. In other words, emotionally, you have to perform at your best so that these other roles are not compromised. The five roles do not require an equal investment of time, but do require an equal investment of your emotional energy. If you have a flat tire on your training ride, just think of all the things you will do to get it fixed before your next ride. That same emotional commitment needs to be made if anything in your five roles needs fixing too.

It's important to be able to understand when your body is telling you that you have had enough physically and emotionally. That something is out of balance. When I was living in Lakewood Ranch and training a lot, I always felt really good. One afternoon I was supposed to go swim, but I just didn't want to. I was tired and wanted to hang out with my kids. I got in the car and started driving to the pool, and then started crying because I didn't want to go, but my mind said, "You have to do this!" In the parking lot of the pool, I sat and asked myself, "What am I doing?" I turned around and went home because I recognized I was out of balance.

-Heather Gollnick

Look at the following graph (Figure 15). On the vertical axis is your EQ Thermometer with GREEN being at the top. On the horizontal axis is the time of day sequenced in three-hour increments.

Think of your day yesterday from the time you woke up till you went to bed. Think of where you were, what you were doing, and most importantly, how you felt at that time (GREEN, YELLOW or RED). At each three-hour mark for the whole day yesterday, put an "X" on how you felt on the vertical axis, based on your EQ temperature.

Feeling great!

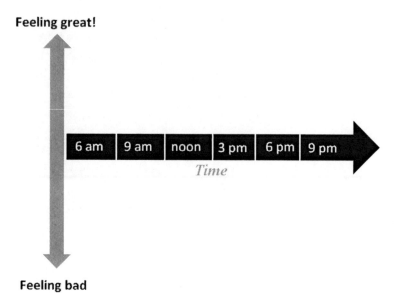

Feeling bad

Figure 15. Monitoring EQ Day

For most people, there will be some highs and lows depending on how your day went. You can do this same exercise for the previous week, month, year, or past 10 or 20 years by just changing the units of the horizontal axis.

Note: It can be a very powerful exercise to do this exercise for your entire life. Have your time line in increments of 5 years to your present age. Plot "X" to the points in your life that were high and low with a one-word descriptor for each one. Refer to the exercise you did in Chapter 2 for experiences in your negative memory bank. Once you do this, you may find a correlation between the events of your low points and the negative monologues you tend to have.

What is important to note is that each day you are likely to be in all colors. This is perfectly normal, and quite frankly, a sign of being emotionally healthy. But if you have to make an important decision, or have to have an important conversation, or be present for an important event for the other roles in your life, when do you think, based on your completed EQ graph of your day yesterday, would have been the best time to do this? Clearly, it would have been when you were GREEN. That is when, from a neuroscience perspective, you feel least threatened, and have full uninhibited access to all your skills and memories – stuff that you will need to be at your best for the important conversation, decision, or event.

This is a key point in having a balance in your life. Balance is not about quantity of time you spend in each role, but the quality of time. Knowing that as a triathlete, a huge chunk of your time will be diverted to your training, it is all the more important to monitor your EQ temperature day by day and make sure you are fully GREEN in the other roles you play, especially when important events in those roles need you to be GREEN.

> I was training a CEO for an Ironman while his wife was pregnant with their fourth child. She was irate. "I need you around – I need help with the kids." He was in charge of the company so he had control over his schedule. I had him schedule his long bike ride for Wednesday mornings. Friday mornings he scheduled a long run. Weekends were freed up. The family was more content and she even started playing tennis on Saturdays with a group of women after the baby. We had arranged his schedule so Saturday's was a short a.m. session and Sundays off for family time. It's all about BALANCE. When the family wanted to go on a ski trip we tweaked his schedule so that his big training week was done before their departure. There is a way to work things out and taking the time and attention to make it work pays great benefits.
>
> -Heather Gollnick

"A man who dares to waste one hour of time has not discovered the value of life." - Charles Darwin

If you have had a bad workout, or a bad day in one of the roles, we do not recommend you "fake" being in GREEN and show up in your other roles with a fake smile, for example. Those that know you well will see right through it. What you need to do is to use your EQ strategy, in much the same way as you would if you had a flat tire on race-day and knowing now that how you respond to it is more important than the mishap itself, as shown in the difference between how Chrissie Wellington and Norman Stadler responded to the same situation. In this context, a triathlon is a wonderful metaphor of life itself. And this just may be the allure of it all, and the answer to why triathlon is both one of the fastest growing sports for middle-aged people, and why they can be addictive.

Life's Mishaps

In the next year, just as in a race, life too will have some mishaps. If they occur in any of the roles that are most important to you, then, just as in a triathlon, have a plan for them.

Exercise: Life's Mishaps

Make a list of 10 life's mishaps that could happen to you in the next 12 months ONLY in the roles in your EQ universe. (Note – if mishaps happen outside of those roles, you do not need to list them here). For each one, think of a solution. Then, as part of making sure you have a balanced life optimizing your happiness, think through by discussing with people in those roles what your solution will be.

1. Mishap:

   _____

   _____

   Solution: _____

   _____

   _____

2. Mishap:

   _____

   _____

   Solution: _____

   _____

   _____

3. Mishap:

   _____

   _____

Solution: _____

_____

4. Mishap:

_____

_____

Solution: _____

_____

_____

5. Mishap:

_____

_____

Solution: _____

_____

_____

6. Mishap:

_____

_____

Solution: _____

_____

_____

7. Mishap:

_____

_____

Solution: _____

_____

_____

8. Mishap:

_____

_____

Solution: _____

_____

_____

9. Mishap:

_____

_____

Solution: _____

_____

_____

10. Mishap:

_____

_____

Solution: _____

_____

"Every man dies. Not every man really lives." - William Wallace

We hope that this book has been a journey of learning for you. One that takes the wonderful sport of triathlon and brings out the best in you. Training to be your best on race-day is the same as training to be your best in life. Now, what could be better?

Top 3 Ideas
I learned from this chapter

1.

2.

3.

3 Action Steps
I will take immediately to incorporate the
above learning for a more balanced life

1.

2.

3.

Chapter Summary

1. Happy athletes tend to be more focused, be able to find focus when it is not there, and perform more consistently at higher levels than those that are not happy.

2. Take the time to properly analyze your life and situation so that you can achieve balance and happiness both in your personal life and with your training.

3. Just as in a race, life, too, will have some mishaps. If they occur in any of the roles that are most important to you, then, just as in a triathlon, have a plan for them.

Last Exercise

The beginning of each chapter in this book is an excerpt from a professional triathlete. Go back and read each one of them. As you read them a second time around, highlight the concepts in this book that they are actually using. For example, highlight in their statement where you notice macro or micro focus, EQ or Skill focal thought, a concerted effort to practice for mishaps, and so on and so forth. You will find the structure we have provided in this book for you is tried and tested by the best athletes in the world.

CPSIA information can be obtained at www.ICGtesting.com
Printed in the USA
BVOW07s1840030813

327647BV00001B/1/P